To past patients, with whom I have learned about chronic fatigue.

To current patients, who have been kind enough to share their journeys toward recovery with me.

To future patients, in anticipation of good outcomes.

May you all enjoy improved health, and may you all be aware of how grateful I am to you for sharing your lives with me.

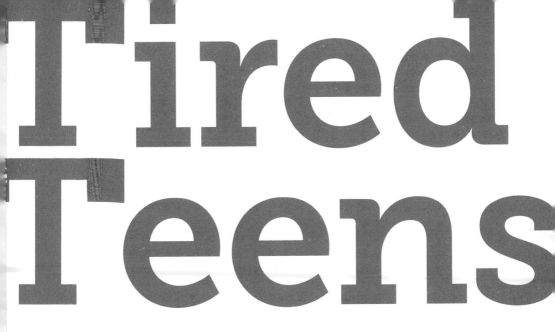

Tired Teens

UNDERSTANDING AND CONQUERING CHRONIC FATIGUE AND POTS

by
Philip R. Fischer, M.D.

with contributions from
Shelley P. Ahrens, APRN, C.N.P., D.N.P.
Laura M. Barron, former patient, medical student
Greg and Shona Barron, Laura's parents
Jeannie E. Clark, R.N.
Kay M. Comisky, R.N.

Published by Mayo Clinic Press

Cover Image: shutterstock411563740.jpg/Credit: © Shutterstock

The information in this book is true and complete to the best of our knowledge. This book is intended as an informative guide for those wishing to learn more about health issues. It is not intended to replace, countermand or conflict with advice given to you by your own physician. The ultimate decision concerning your care should be made between you and your doctor. Information in this book if offered with no guarantees. The author and publisher disclaim all liability in connection with the use of this book. The views expressed are the author's personal views, and do not necessarily reflect the policy or position of Mayo Clinic.

For bulk sales to employers, member groups and health-related companies, contact Mayo Clinic, 200 First St. SW, Rochester, MN 55905, call 800-430-9699, or send an email to *SpecialSalesMayoBooks@mayo.edu.*

ISBN 978-1-893005-65-5

Library of Congress Control Number: 2020945786

Printed in the United States of America

Welcome, readers!

I, my family, thousands of tired teenagers, and this book have grown up together.

Personally, I was down with chronic post-infectious fatigue when my third child was born three decades ago. I was recovering when my fourth child was born. That fourth child did a high school science project about postural orthostatic tachycardia syndrome (POTS) several years ago and then became the father of a daughter on the same day that the proof copy of this book was delivered to me.

Through generations, children grow through adolescence into adulthood, sometimes with debilitating fatigue along the way. Yet, there is always hope of recovery and of new birth. From my personal and professional experiences, this book has been "born" and is now delivered to you.

I offer this book with the hope that it will encourage and inspire you as you face chronic fatigue in yourself or in someone about whom you care deeply. I give you these words and pages in expectation that you, too, will find healing and recovery. I am eager to see and hear about how your recoveries will allow you to grow and serve others. May this book help overcome illness, restore health, provide hope, and generate life-enhancing productivity.

Share your stories and ideas with me at *TiredTeenagers@gmail.com*. Enjoy!

Phil Fischer

Table of Contents

Acknowledgments

It has been 15 years since this book was initially conceived, and it has been over a decade since the actual drafting of a manuscript began. I am very grateful to many key individuals who have been instrumental in making this book available to readers. A high school writing teacher, the late Rod Flagler, inspired a passion for writing within me. Fred Glauser ignited my passion for medical research. Chris Frye and Neil Gudovitz helped turn ideas about tired teenagers into a book proposal. Olivia Smoldt-Hall provided professional expertise in molding my writing style into more engaging prose. Rachel Haring Bartony, along with Dan Harke and Karen Wallevand at Mayo Clinic Press, skillfully turned my initial faltering drafts into the book you see before you now.

Shelley Ahrens has shared patients with me and contributed greatly to the actual writing of this manuscript. The contributions of Laura and her parents brought this book to life, with hope and healing for readers; now Laura is doing high-level research about the anatomy and physiology of brain connectivity in patients with POTS and pain. Jeannie Clark, Kay Comisky, Amy Belal, and Meg Steuer help our shared patients make practical steps toward recovery, and I am grateful for Jeannie's and Kay's tangible contributions to this book.

Along the way, I have learned from and with Co-Burn Porter, Dawn Nelson, Chad Brands, Jon Caudill, Karen Ytterberg, Anne Jones, Kelsey Klaas, Mike Farrell, and many others in Rochester, Minnesota. Our ongoing research and patient care at Mayo Clinic is helped by subspecialty colleagues, including Ken Mack, Sheri Driscoll, Cindy Harbeck-Weber, Bridget Biggs, Daniel Hilliker, Tracy Harrison, Bob Wilder, Louai Manini, Robin Lloyd, and the rest of our Mayo Clinic Adolescent Autonomic Dysfunction Working Group (generously supported by the Greg and Beth Wahl family).

I have benefited from professional friendships with co-laborers in the conquest to overcome chronic fatigue around the world — Nelly Ninis, Raewyn Gavin, Nancy Kuntz, Julian Stewart, Marvin Medow, Gisela and Tom Chelimsky, Imad Jarjour, Paul Pianosi, Mohammed Numan, and many others in the pediatric group within the American Autonomic Society.

I have been blessed by the help of Debbie Dominelli at Dysautonomia Youth Network of America and have enjoyed collaboration with the Freemans at The Dysautonomia Project and Lauren Stiles at Dysautonomia International. Julie and Gil Chinitz and American Dysautonomia Institute have been helpfully supportive over the years. Lesley Kavi and the whole POTS UK group have taught me lots, too. And "adult" colleagues who know lots more about POTS than I do have helped me along the way — Phillip Low, Wolfgang Singer, Paola Sandroni, and others at Mayo Clinic and through the American Autonomic Society with people like Bill Cheshire and Satish Raj. Robin Youngson from Hearts in Healthcare and friends in the Paediatric Society of New Zealand helped refine my thoughts about caring for tired teenagers.

Positive value from the content of this book is due to the helpful input and influence of these and many other key professionals; problems in the book are my responsibility, and I'd like to hear about them so they can be corrected if there is a subsequent edition of this book.

Personally, patients and coworkers have been my extended family over the years. But I am fundamentally grateful for and indebted to my wife, Juli, and our five children, two daughters-in-law, and now four grandchildren for their support, help, and encouragement throughout this long process. Mostly, though, I attribute whatever hope and healing this book provides for tired teenagers and their families to the grace and power of God who makes all things possible.

To all, thanks very much.

Preface

Teenagers are tired.

In near-epidemic proportions, adolescents today are struggling with fatigue.

Teenagers know this. Many hit the snooze button and delay getting out of bed for as long as possible in the morning. They're still dragging when they get to school, and they use caffeinated drinks to help them get through the morning.

Parents know teens are tired. They struggle to encourage their kids to get up and get ready for school, but they feel like they're nagging. Then long after their own bedtime, parents try to convince their teenagers to go to bed so parents won't be so tired in the morning.

Schools know teenagers are tired. Some have even tried shifting to a later morning start time. Teachers recognize that adolescent academic performance improves midmorning.

And doctors know teenagers are tired. Research suggests that close to a third of American adolescent girls struggle with morning fatigue more than once a week. In Europe, about 20% of Dutch girls and 7% of Dutch boys struggle with tiredness that has persisted for more than three months. In England, more than one out of every 100 adolescents is disabled with fatigue and unable to participate in regular school and social activities.

Fatigue is common, and it messes up lives. All over the world, teenagers and their families struggle with fatigue. Unfortunately, neither the teenagers nor their parents understand why teens are so tired, and their doctors have struggled unsuccessfully to give them clear answers.

Why are so many teenagers tired?

Is there an underlying "mystery diagnosis" robbing adolescents of energy?

How can they recover?

You see, I'm a pediatrician, and I care for patients who travel up to thousands of miles to find answers and to begin recovery. Many of my patients are tired, and they haven't started getting better despite even years of good motivation and dedicated effort by themselves, by their families, and by their doctors. Most of the people we see end up finding answers, hope, and healing. This is good, but the word has spread. Hundreds of families want to come see the team with which I work, but we can't grow our staff fast enough to see all the people who want to come for help.

So I'm writing this book as a personal message to you, whether you're a tired teen or the loved one of a tired teen. My goal is to help you find direction in your quest for recovery. My goal is to provide you with answers and with the tools to help you actually get better. I'd love to meet you and to work with you personally, but I'd love it even more if you could recover without needing to see us.

Even though this book is intended as a personal communication with you, it has taken a huge team to allow me to provide these pages. I had lots of great teachers over the years, and I've learned even more from patients and families since completing my pediatric training in 1984. Great colleagues have participated in this journey to understand chronic fatigue in adolescents. We don't have all the answers yet, but science has advanced enough to provide lots of help. It's taken time and the help of many people to bring this book to you.

Still, recovery won't come simply by reading this book or even by implementing the suggestions on these pages. You'll need your own team to foster recovery. Your team will include supportive family and friends, caring health professionals, and a whole host of other people. I hope that the words of this book will provide enough information and even inspiration to help you get started down a successful road to recovery.

It's miserable to feel tired! Many other teens are struggling with fatigue also. You'll get through this difficult journey. The tiredness and misery aren't permanent.

What this book is about

This book is about tired teenagers. It's about why they're tired and how they can recover. What can you anticipate as you read? The first two sections deal with persistent fatigue in general and can help you understand why you feel tired and what you can do about it. The third and fourth sections are dedicated specifically to teens whose chronic fatigue is part of a condition known as postural orthostatic tachycardia syndrome (POTS). POTS accounts for more than half of the disabling fatigue in teens.

Who this book is for

So who might benefit from this book? You — if you're an adolescent bothered by long-term fatigue. You — if you have a family member or friend suffering from bothersome tiredness. You — if you provide care to tired teenagers. Sometimes, comments are mostly directed to teens, and at other times comments are useful mostly for friends and relatives of tired teens. But we all benefit together as we share information. My hope is that every reader will find value in this book, and that ultimately these pages will help tired teens and their families make progress to real recovery.

We're in this together. I'll share my years of experience treating teens with fatigue, while one of my former patients, Laura, and her parents will discuss the more personal side of living with POTS and chronic fatigue. Later, I'll share insights from some of our nurses, Jeannie and Kay, too. Now, though, let's hear from Laura.

👤 LAURA

I led a normal, healthy life growing up. As a competitive swimmer and violinist, I was always on the go; a normal day for me involved rushing from a full day at school to a 3-hour swim practice, followed by a violin lesson, dinner, homework, and sleep. I loved being busy and doing the things I enjoyed. So when I got sick at the age of 15, it was devastating. At first, I simply felt sluggish in the water — not performing to my level of ability. Then other symptoms started to arise — a racing heart rate, chronic headaches, nausea, and extreme fatigue. Over a period of three months, I went from training three to six hours a day to barely being able to walk up a flight of stairs. I could not drag myself out of bed in the morning, and would sleep the whole day away. I was unrecognizable from the lively, active teenager I had been just months before. My family and I went from doctor to doctor, trying to find an answer for what was happening to me. No matter how many tests were run, no one could seem to find a concrete diagnosis, and I became increasingly frustrated as I watched life go by from my bed.

In retrospect, many of the early signs were evident that would have indicated that Laura was beginning to struggle with POTS. The problem was that we had no idea what was happening. Laura had been a competitive swimmer for years. During the summer between her freshman and sophomore years of high school she was participating in swim team practices twice a day. While her teammates were going to movies, working, or hanging out between practice sessions, our daughter was sleeping. She would complain of her feet and legs feeling so "heavy." Despite the twice-a-day practices and her long periods of rest, her racing swim times got slower and slower. She looked very pale and her energy level was best described as sluggish. She was just 15 years old.

As parents we just thought she was training too hard and likely growing, which was putting a significant amount of stress on her body. So it seemed understandable that she might need more sleep. The first specialist we saw felt her issues were due to overtraining. The treatment was to stop swimming for a month, rest, and focus on nutrition. In the fall of her junior year, she continued to slide further and further until the fatigue kept her from attending school regularly. All the while we were going from doctor to doctor to determine the cause of her ever-increasing number of symptoms. All the test results were coming back as normal but the symptoms persisted.

It took a while for our daughter to develop the dizziness, tachycardia [rapid heart rate], and severe brain fog. Once she stopped swimming and was spending the majority of her time sleeping, she became more and more deconditioned and the symptoms came on full force. Unfortunately the symptoms were coming fast and furious but the test results never changed.

They remained normal. We still did not have a diagnosis. Our now 16-year-old daughter was sleeping about 20 hours a day and she was miserable. Our happy-go-lucky, sweet and energetic daughter was gone and we began to fear that she might not get better. Her life looked nothing like it did one year before. Simple tasks like getting out of bed, showering, and getting dressed were major hurdles. She was spinning out of control, and we were beyond worried and very frightened. Without a diagnosis, we were losing hope and frustrated, as no one could help us understand what was happening.

So, you've met me, and now you've met Laura and her parents. Along the way, you'll hear more from all of us, and you'll also get to read comments from Jeannie and Kay, great nurses who have helped hundreds of teenagers overcome POTS and other forms of chronic fatigue. Ultimately, I look forward to hearing stories of your full and complete recovery from fatigue. (Write to me at *TiredTeenagers@ gmail.com.*)

Misery and hope. Tiredness and recovery. There is potential that each of you and the people for whom you care can be accurately diagnosed and that you can actually get better. Recovery? Yes, full recovery is possible.

ⓘ SOME IMPORTANT DEFINITIONS

Before we move forward, let's make sure we're talking the same language. Let's review some definitions. These definitions will introduce some topics to frame ongoing discussions, and I'll talk about all of this in more detail later.

Fatigue. Practically, we can consider the terms *fatigue* and *tiredness* to mean the same thing. While sleepiness can be part of fatigue and tiredness, in this book we usually take fatigue and tiredness to mean more than just sleepiness, and to indicate a generalized sense of lacking energy. It can feel like a heaviness of both body and mind. It can feel like a burden that makes activity seem overwhelmingly difficult.

Chronic. The word *chronic* means long-term. Usually, fatigue is considered to be chronic when it has persisted for three or more months. And chronic fatigue implies that the fatigue is almost always present, as opposed to intermittent fatigue, which comes and goes. Chronic fatigue can rise and fall in intensity, but it's usually felt almost all of the time.

Syndrome. The term *syndrome* refers to a collection of symptoms or physical findings that fit together. For example, POTS is a syndrome associated with a set of specific symptoms that you'll learn about later.

Autonomic nervous system. The involuntary (autonomic) nervous system regulates things we don't usually need to think about. It controls blood flow, intestinal flow, and temperature, among other things.

Autonomic dysfunction. Sometimes, the involuntary nervous system gets out of balance, and people have trouble with blood flow (dizziness, fatigue), intestinal flow (nausea, abdominal discomfort), or temperature regulation (feeling hotter or colder than peers, having sensations like hot flashes). We call this situation autonomic dysfunction, and some people use the similar term *dysautonomia*. Autonomic dysfunction can be a problem in and of itself, or it can stem from a separate medical problem that reveals itself through the autonomic nervous system.

Orthostatic intolerance. Some tired adolescents, like Laura, have extreme fatigue associated with an inability to exercise, as well as bothersome dizziness when standing up. These teenagers often also have headaches and abdominal discomfort. When someone feels worse standing up rather than lying down on a daily basis, we say that the person has orthostatic intolerance. Ortho refers to the upright position, and intolerance means, well, that the person doesn't tolerate the position very well.

Postural orthostatic tachycardia syndrome (POTS). POTS is a form of autonomic dysfunction characterized by long-term orthostatic intolerance and an excessive change in heart rate when switching to an upright position. Some people have just autonomic dysfunction with orthostatic intolerance — very similar to the symptoms of POTS. But people with POTS also have an excessive change in heart rate when they stand up. Some people, like Laura, notice that their hearts race when standing up, or their doctors notice this. The term *postural* relates to position change, the term *orthostatic* refers to being upright and still, and the term *tachycardia* means fast heart. The term *syndrome* indicates a collection of symptoms such as long-term fatigue, daily trouble being upright, excessive heart rate when standing up, and other symptoms like headache and abdominal discomfort. For simplicity, some people leave the word *orthostatic* out of the label and refer to the condition as postural tachycardia syndrome.

CHRONIC FATIGUE VS. CHRONIC FATIGUE SYNDROME

Sometimes chronic fatigue is also referred to as a syndrome. When I use the term *chronic fatigue* in this book, I'm referring to a long-term experience of tiredness and lack of energy. People who have chronic fatigue often have lots of other symptoms, and these other symptoms sometimes make up a specific cluster that's shared by other people. Since the 1990s, researchers have lumped several symptoms and findings together into what's called chronic fatigue syndrome. This sort of clustering can be useful in research studies, to make sure that study participants are actually similar and comparable. But in common usage, the term *chronic fatigue syndrome* has sometimes come to mean a tiredness associated with lots of other problems that aren't well understood and from which you might never recover. So I don't like to use the chronic fatigue syndrome label outside of research settings since it ends up discouraging patients and their families unnecessarily. As you will see in this book, we actually do understand a lot about chronic fatigue, and most people do get better.

👥 LAURA'S PARENTS

A few months after Laura's 16th birthday we made our way to the Mayo Clinic in Rochester, Minnesota, where we finally determined what was happening. Finally, a diagnosis! We were very relieved to have a treatment plan and were hopeful that Laura's recovery journey would begin.

Ready? We've set the stage. We've connected with Laura and her parents. We understand some important terms. We want to overcome chronic fatigue. Now, let's get moving!

Section 1: Chronic fatigue

Chapter 1: Got sleep?

It takes effort to enjoy winter in Minnesota. It's dark when I go to work, and it's dark again before I head home. The air is frigidly cold and walkways are icy. In southern California where I grew up, the weather almost always seemed perfect. After 22 Minnesota winters, though, I feel a bit sorry for people stuck in California. They miss out on seasons. Californians don't get to enjoy lawns covered with fall leaves and the springtime return of migrating birds.

Our world was created with rhythms and patterns. The seasons change. The sun rises and sets. The rhythms of human life, such as our music and our sports, in many ways reflect the changing cycles of the natural world. We prefer rhythms to monotone music, and we like both pauses and crescendos. Our sports contests have quarters and innings and periods, and each sport has its season. We move from one phase of activity to the next.

Our bodies, too, were designed to follow rhythms. Our body chemistry and our hormones follow cycling patterns. We rest and rejuvenate at night, and we actively deplete our stored resources during the day. We cycle between activity and rest, from times of energy expenditure to periods of recovery.

Except when we're busy.

Sometimes, feeling tired all day is simply a matter of not getting enough sleep. We may think that what we're doing is so important or we allow our lives to get so busy that we don't have time to slow down and let our bodies go through the rest cycles for which they were designed.

Sleep needs

A while ago, a young teen came from a few states away to see me because she was tired all the time. After a thorough evaluation, I realized that her only problem was that she wasn't getting enough sleep. I explained that the average adolescent needs about nine hours of sleep each night and that her six hours simply weren't enough. Her mother stiffened up, raised her voice, and exclaimed that "You don't understand teenagers in Texas. She's too busy to get more than six hours of sleep each night." Clearly, this mother and daughter had unrealistic expectations about what a body can do and how much sleep is actually necessary.

In the United States, high schoolers get an average of seven and a half hours of sleep each night. Sure, some bodies are set up to do fine with this, but others need more than the average nine hours per night. Insufficient sleep contributes to lots of fatigue. While each person is an individual, most adolescents need nine hours of good sleep each night.

What makes us think we're too busy to sleep?

For some teens — high-achieving gymnasts and dancers, for example — there's this notion that you need to practice a sport for four to six hours per day and excel at schoolwork and spend lots of time with friends. Adolescent bodies are rarely prepared to perform at professional levels while maintaining other normal teen life activities.

Other teenagers have become "possessed" by their possessions. One of the hardest struggles for people when dealing with a severe storm is to go without electricity. They have no way to charge their phones and other devices. Similarly, technology tools that were designed to help us can end up enslaving us. We begin to think we need to be turned on and logged in and responding to others 24 hours a day.

For years, we have known that watching too much television leads to obesity and fatigue. Wise pediatric leaders suggest that adolescents spend no more than two hours per day watching screens — television, videos, movies, social media, noneducational internet sites. Nonetheless, most teenagers spend at least twice that much time each day in front of a screen! Do you sleep with your cell phone in your hand? It could be that you and your phone are not allowing your body to relax enough to get into the good deep sleep stages. Sometimes we get "too busy" doing things that seem normal even though they work against our physical and mental health.

Lots of things can make us think we're too busy to get enough sleep — whether sports or schoolwork or just hanging with friends. Each of us needs to set priorities. Once we're out of balance and getting tired, though, we start doing things less comfortably and less effectively. That's when it might be appropriate to do a time inventory and clean up our schedule so that we're balancing important things with adequate time to relax and sleep. We need breaks and changes of scenery during the day. Perhaps that should include some "technology fasts" where we go without direct connection with our communication devices.

Are you getting enough sleep? If you use an alarm to wake up, your body is probably not adequately rested. If you sleep longer on weekends than during the week, then your body is probably trying to "pay back" the "sleep debt" that accumulated during the week. Either way, you probably need more sleep!

No amount of sleep seemed to alleviate my overwhelming fatigue. I frequently slept the day away, and would start feeling more awake by the late afternoon and into the evening. When it was actually time for me to go to bed for the night, I would feel wide awake, even though I was still extremely fatigued. My sleep hygiene at this time was dismal. I would watch TV in bed when I could not fall asleep, and always had my phone right next to me throughout the night.

Sleep and the rhythms of life

How does sleep work, anyway?

In Alaska, where I "hid" to finish writing this book, bears shut down for the winter. They put their bodies into slow motion as a means of surviving until more food becomes available. Humans don't hibernate. We don't really shut down at night. Instead, we keep burning energy, about 90% to 95% of our daytime level of energy consumption. Instead of turning off, our brains cycle through a series of sleep stages. Our hormone levels go up and down. Our muscles relax. Our circulation clears excess waste from our systems. Our bodies rejuvenate and grow. Human sleep isn't simply like the inactivity of a hibernating bear. Rather, sleep is a programmed series of restorative events.

Studies of human brain waves identify several different stages of sleep. When you drift off to sleep, your brain gradually shifts into progressively deeper phases of sleep called non-rapid eye movement (NREM) sleep. In the deepest phase of sleep, brain waves are large and slow, and you're more difficult to awaken. This is the most restorative phase of sleep. From deep sleep, you move into rapid eye movement or REM sleep, during which the eyes move and the body is relatively paralyzed. Dreams take place during the REM phase. For older teens and adults, the body cycles through NREM and then REM sleep about every 90 minutes, and later night sleep is richer in the REM component. Disruption of these cycles can lead to trouble during the day, including the inability to focus and perform mental tasks.

Awakening is most effective when people wake up during light sleep, such as just after completing a whole sleep cycle terminating with full REM sleep. Rather than waking up according to a time on a clock, some people are now buying alarm clocks that sense their sleep stage and awaken them during light sleep.

Daytime napping sometimes provides an escape to help stave off some sleepiness. But it doesn't allow for bodily restoration like full nighttime sleep cycles do. And daytime napping makes it harder to initiate sleep at an appropriate time.

A 2005 report in the medical journal *Pediatrics* suggested that 15 million American children were not getting enough sleep. Things haven't improved much since then. And the sleepless teenagers in that study had more health problems and less family harmony at home than did those teens who got enough sleep. American children and adolescents need more sleep, and they need better sleep.

⏱ QUICK TAKE

So what does all this mean? First, people will be most refreshed and least fatigued if they get enough sleep. For most teenagers, enough is about nine hours each night. Second, sleep is most useful if it's allowed to cycle through all stages and if awakening occurs after completing deeper sleep followed by a complete REM stage. Waking up to an alarm clock determined by a schedule is less effective than timing day-night cycles to allow for spontaneous morning awakening. Third, naps are okay for emergencies, but frequent naps end up leading to lower quality and quantity of necessary nighttime sleep.

Regulating sleep cycles

The daily cycle of wakefulness and sleep is called the circadian rhythm. One of the key physiologic factors regulating sleep is a chemical called melatonin. Melatonin is secreted during the evening from the pineal gland in the head. Melatonin helps to initiate sleep in the evening and maintain sleep through the night. We know that teenagers often go through changes in their circadian rhythms. Often, they end up shifting their natural sleep cycles so they start sleep later in the evening and don't feel like waking up until later in the morning.

✚ NOTES FROM A NURSE

The combination of teens and routine isn't the norm but it must be to facilitate recovery. Humans naturally are attracted to what feels good and are more likely to choose what feels good over what doesn't. Unfortunately, when we commit to balance, our choices include not only what feels good but also what is beneficial yet difficult. Meeting a challenge is what builds resilience and molds us as we experience life.

Teens' brains are even more susceptible to being drawn to pleasure. Their brains default to choosing what feels good and what is immediate. This is why human children live with their parents for so many years. (I remember living with my parents and thinking, "Wow, I know more than my parents. I am only still here because I cannot afford to be on my own.") The brain of a growing teen needs to continue to develop until the teen can be safely independent.

Parents are there to help guide their children and encourage them to follow through with those not-so-pleasurable choices or experiences, thus helping to build resiliency and success.

— Kay

External influencers of sleep

There are several external factors that also affect circadian rhythm and sleep effectiveness.

Light exposure Darkness stimulates melatonin release, and exposure to light reduces melatonin levels. It's helpful to dim lights before bedtime and sleep in a dark area. It's also helpful not to look at a lighted screen for at least an hour before trying to fall asleep.

Stimulants Stimulants like caffeine and attention deficit medications (and illicit substances like cocaine) charge the brain up in a way that makes sleep difficult. Depressants like alcohol and marijuana might make people feel a bit sleepier, but they also reduce the amount and effectiveness of REM sleep with a net effect of worsening overall sleep.

Physical activity Exercise should be part of a daily activity-sleep cycle. However, exercise keeps a body revved up temporarily and can make sleep initiation more difficult for about two hours after physical activity. Thus, exercise is important, but it is most effective if completed well before bedtime.

Schedules Some school districts are shifting start times to allow "night owls" to get plenty of sleep before getting up to start the next day. Even professional pediatric and sleep medicine groups advocate for later morning starts to adolescent school days. In other areas, teenagers can adjust their evening schedules — such as exercising earlier in the day if possible, avoiding stimulants in the late afternoon or evening hours, shutting down devices, and darkening the bedroom before bedtime — to help shift their circadian rhythms to promote earlier sleep initiation. Whatever mental and physical activity will be required during the day, the mind will be sharper and the body readier if sleep has been adequate.

👥 LAURA'S PARENTS

Our daughter was extremely sensitive to light when she was trying to sleep. Even a small night light or the light from her alarm clock was enough to interfere with her ability to relax into sleep and to stay asleep. She had a blackout blind in her bedroom, which made the room very dark, and that seemed to help with this light issue. Additionally, Laura had severe noise sensitivity that would disrupt her sleep. Her solution for this issue was a small floor fan in her room that generated constant white noise. To this day, when our daughter comes home to visit, the blind is down, the nightlight is unplugged, the alarm clock is covered, and the fan is going in her bedroom.

Sleep disorders

In addition to poor sleep habits, there are several common sleep disorders that lead to inadequate sleep and excessive fatigue. Warning signs of these sleep problems should prompt a visit with your doctor. Appropriate medical care can improve sleep and decrease fatigue.

Restless legs syndrome This condition is seen in about one in 50 teenagers, but it often gets missed and remains undiagnosed. About two-thirds of teenagers with restless legs syndrome have a close relative with the same condition even though it is often un-diagnosed in the relative, too.

People with restless legs syndrome notice discomfort in their legs, especially around bedtime. This discomfort can be anything from growing pain-type achiness to tingling or electrical shooting pains. The discomfort is relieved to some degree by moving the legs, and people with restless legs syndrome are often tired during the day since they don't sleep well at night.

Formal sleep studies would show abnormally frequent limb movements during sleep, but the diagnosis is usually made by the physician, who notes the restlessness, discomfort, and poor sleep. Lack of iron can sometimes cause or aggravate restless legs syndrome. Initial treatment is usually with iron to get the iron stores up above the range where many people keep them (a ferritin level of at least 50 nanograms per milliliter, or ng/mL). Other neurological medications also can be effective if needed.

Obstructive sleep apnea Sometimes snoring is a sign of obstruction in the throat — either by big tonsils or adenoids or both, or by weakness or floppiness of the throat tissues. Medical evaluation is warranted for a teenager with fatigue who snores.

Sometimes, the brain arouses frequently during the night (even without the person being aware) as the snorer pauses breathing and then gasps to catch a breath. Doctors call this condition obstructive sleep apnea. This interrupts the regular cycling of sleep stages and leaves the individual unrefreshed in the morning and tired throughout much of the day. Treatment depends on the cause and varies from tonsil removal to using a pressure machine (continuous positive airway pressure or CPAP) to help keep the airway open at night.

Depression and anxiety

People with depression, anxiety, or both have alterations in their brain chemicals. One of these chemicals is serotonin. Adequately regulated serotonin is needed to produce the right amount of melatonin to help sleep. Tired teenagers with poor sleep and any hint of mood problems should see a doctor to make sure that anxiety and depression aren't going untreated. Whether poor sleep caused mood troubles or whether mood troubles caused poor sleep, every aspect of the tired teenager should be treated.

Truly, there are many factors contributing to adolescent fatigue. For many affected teens, though, inadequate sleep is part of the problem — either not enough time sleeping or not enough high-quality sleep when they are sleeping. Adjusting evening schedules, avoiding sleep-altering chemicals, and disconnecting from technology can help improve sleep for some people. And some tired teenagers need medical intervention for underlying conditions such as restless legs syndrome, obstructive sleep apnea, or mood disorders.

Chapter 2:
I'm tired because
I'm sick

Is there a doctor in the house? My own children tend to go online to MayoClinic.org rather than come to me when they have health questions. Whether we believe our parents or the internet, we do need to consider different diseases and diagnoses as we deal with fatigue.

In addition to the lifestyle factors and sleep disorders I've already discussed, lots of other problems can cause fatigue. Thus, it's important for teens with significant fatigue to talk to a doctor. Here are other treatable medical conditions that can cause intermittent or persistent fatigue.

Iron deficiency and anemia

A 12-year-old patient of mine began to experience fatigue while vacationing in Europe. Even though she wanted to look through museums and visit shops and restaurants, she was too tired to walk that much. After missing out on lots of the activities planned during her trip, she saw a doctor and learned she was anemic. Anemia is where you have a lower-than-normal amount and concentration of red blood cells in your circulation system. Red blood cells carry oxygen to different tissues to support the body's production and use of energy.

Identifying anemia, however, isn't the end of a medical evaluation. The cause of anemia also needs to be determined. This traveling 12-year-old had overly heavy periods and didn't eat much meat. She was iron deficient and got better with iron supplementation. I know another adolescent who was chronically tired — she had anemia that turned out to be due to leukemia. She also got better with treatment.

Some fatigue results from iron deficiency even without anemia. Any adolescent with significant fatigue should have blood tests to rule out anemia and to check ferritin levels to make sure there's no iron deficiency present. Ferritin is a measure of stored reserves of iron. Even if there's no anemia but iron deficiency is identified, the iron deficiency should be treated.

Hormone issues

Hormones are chemical messengers. They travel from one part of the body to another in order to communicate how various body parts should be functioning. Some deal with general body functions like metabolism, and others deal with more-specific body functions, like growth and puberty and urine production.

Thyroid disorders People vary in terms of how they burn off (metabolize) energy. Part of the body's metabolism is controlled by the thyroid gland in the neck. People who are low on thyroid hormones tend to feel sluggish. They also tend to gain weight, get constipated, and have decreased knee reflexes (the kind of reflex your doctor tests with a slight tap to the knee). Most tired teenagers should probably have their thyroid function checked with a blood test.

There are several possible blood tests for thyroid function. The test for thyroid-stimulating hormone (TSH) — the stuff produced in the pituitary part of the brain that tells the thyroid gland in the neck how hard to work — is the best test. If the test result is too high (more than 10 milli-international units per liter, or mIU/L), the patient has a low-functioning thyroid (hypothyroidism) that is probably contributing to the fatigue.

Treatment with oral thyroid hormones can help. If the TSH level is just a little high (between 5 and 10 mIU/L), thyroid function can be monitored with repeated blood tests to make sure a thyroid problem isn't developing. It's unlikely, though, that mild thyroid abnormalities (with TSH levels less than 10) are the main cause of the fatigue. Some medical professionals argue that even TSH levels between 3 and 5 mIU/L are too high, but there isn't good evidence that these levels of TSH are associated with fatigue.

Diabetes Sometimes, but not often, other hormone problems can cause fatigue without a lot of other symptoms. Diabetes occurs when the body doesn't produce enough insulin to appropriately use sugar. Adolescents with diabetes and high blood sugar levels can feel tired, but they usually have other signs of trouble as well — like excessive thirst, excessive urine output, a huge appetite, and weight loss. Nonetheless, it's reasonable for your doctor to check blood sugar or do a urinalysis to make sure there's no evidence of diabetes.

Low blood sugar (hypoglycemia) Low blood sugar levels can cause fatigue. But low blood sugar rarely happens on its own. People with diabetes who get more insulin than they need can have low blood sugar — with fatigue and shakiness and sweatiness at times. People, usually young children, with specific disorders that affect cellular energy output (mitochondrial disorders) can have low blood sugar levels when they go too long without eating. Without another underlying serious disease, though, it's extremely unusual for hypoglycemia by itself to cause chronic fatigue in teenagers.

Adrenal disorders Adrenal glands — small glands located above the kidneys — respond to physical challenges by putting out more steroid hormones. This helps to energize the body. In healthy people, the adrenal hormone cortisol builds up during the night and then gets used up during the day. Overactive adrenal glands that produce too much cortisol make people gain weight and feel "sludgy." Underactive adrenal glands leave people tired, too. An overly high cortisol level in the morning suggests Cushing disease and should prompt additional testing. An excessively low cortisol level in the morning after a good night's rest raises concerns for adrenal insufficiency (Addison disease). Having seen thousands of tired teenagers, though, I know that adrenal disease is very rarely the cause of their fatigue.

Kidney problems

Kidneys filter waste from the body and send it to the bladder to be flushed out as urine. In some children, the urine flows backward from the bladder, and this scars the kidneys. This is usually associated with recurrent urinary tract infections (UTIs), but sometimes can also lead to poor kidney function (seen by elevated levels of creatinine and blood urea nitrogen, or BUN), high blood pressure, and fatigue. Other signs that kidney dysfunction might be underlying fatigue could be excessive blood or protein in the urine. So it makes sense to test for these substances in an adolescent with otherwise unexplained fatigue.

Liver problems

The liver is one of the original recyclers. It was "going green" by producing green bile from waste products long before environmental awareness became prominent. When the liver gets hurt or sick, though, it fails to clear toxic waste from the body, and fatigue can result. Infection with a hepatitis virus can cause fatigue (and usually yellowness, or jaundice, as well). I once treated a girl with fatigue that turned out to be due to autoimmune hepatitis (where the immune system makes antibodies that attack the liver). If a doctor sees a tired teenager and isn't sure what's causing the tiredness, he or she will probably include some liver tests (like the enzyme ALT test) as part of the medical evaluation. As with other tests, abnormal results might not provide the final answer but would prompt the doctor to keep looking for the underlying cause of the liver trouble.

Other digestive troubles

Lots of tired teenagers have belly issues — nausea, discomfort, constipation, or intermittent loose stools. Often, these difficulties are due to whatever else is causing the fatigue rather than a primary gastrointestinal problem. Sometimes, though, trouble with absorbing nutrition does lead to fatigue.

Celiac disease, for example, can cause poor intestinal absorption. Some people are born with genes from one or both parents that predispose them to developing antibodies that attack the lining of the small intestine. The production of these antibodies is stimulated by eating wheat and other gluten-containing foods. This leads to inflammation that thins the intestinal layer where enzymes break down and absorb food. Even without specific gastrointestinal symptoms, some people with early celiac disease just feel tired and yucky. Blood tests can give clues to gluten sensitivity — revealing antibodies or specific genes related to the risk of celiac disease. If these tests suggest possible gluten sensitivity, then a definitive diagnostic test (looking at the intestines through a scope and getting intestinal biopsies) is usually recommended to see if it's necessary to eliminate gluten from the diet.

Inflammatory bowel disease (IBD) is a different intestinal problem. The two main forms are Crohn's disease and ulcerative colitis. Either can present with fatigue, but usually with abdominal pain and bloody stools as well. Blood tests, such as sedimentation rate and C-reactive protein, often reveal increased inflammation in people with IBD. If a person has symptoms suggestive of IBD — and especially if he or she also has otherwise unexplained anemia — then tests such as endoscopy and colonoscopy might be needed to rule out IBD.

Infection

It's easy to try to blame germs for chronic fatigue. The human immunodeficiency virus (HIV) causes acquired immunodeficiency syndrome (AIDS) and can be associated with chronic fatigue.

Chronic infections such as brucellosis and Lyme disease have been thought to cause isolated fatigue. But these conditions are, in fact, fairly easily diagnosable and are fully treatable with standard medical practices. Despite some rumors and myths to the contrary, embarking on prolonged antibiotic therapy for presumed Lyme disease probably doesn't help chronic fatigue and might distract teenagers and their families from finding a more-effective treatment. And long-term antibiotic therapy can cause lots of side effects.

⊙ QUICK TAKE

So, what does all this medical stuff mean? It means that an adolescent with otherwise unexplained fatigue should see his or her doctor for a medical evaluation. The doctor will probably do some basic blood and urine tests to make sure that iron deficiency, anemia, a hormonal imbalance, kidney dysfunction, liver disease, an inflammatory condition, or an infection isn't causing the fatigue. Sometimes a problem will be identified and corrected, and the fatigue will resolve.

For many patients with long-term tiredness, though, all of the blood, urine, imaging, and biopsy tests yield normal results. Even when tiredness is accompanied by other symptoms such as dizziness and nausea, medical tests don't identify specific structural problems in the body. Even in these cases, though, there is room for more discussion, more evaluation, more treatment, and great hope for full recovery.

Section 2: What's happening in the body

Chapter 3: You feel bad but don't know why

Maybe you're approaching your 16th birthday. You'd like to be thinking about getting your driver's license. You should be studying and enjoying extracurricular activities. Instead, you struggle even to go to school. You feel tired all the time but can't sleep well at night. You get dizzy and sometimes can't see for a few seconds when you stand up. Your stomach is uncomfortable, and eating isn't fun. Life seems to be passing you by.

Perhaps, a year and a half ago, you were getting straight As at school while taking advanced classes. You had lots of friends. You were a starter on your school's volleyball team. You sang a solo in the choir's winter concert. Everything seemed perfect — until you got mono (or had an injury like a concussion).

After a week and a half of fevers with a sore throat, you were left feeling wiped out all the time. You tried to go back to school but couldn't last through a whole day. The volleyball season came and went, without you. You were too dizzy to stand up with the choir to practice. The mono (or concussion) is long gone, and your life seems to be fading away as well. The worst part is that you're just not sure why everything seems to be falling apart like it is.

Your doctors have done all sorts of tests. Your thyroid is okay. You're not anemic. Nearly a hundred other tests have come back negative. Your doctor wonders if you're overreacting or just afraid to go to school. You cried when you heard that and never want to see that doctor again.

What's wrong with you?

Maybe this isn't actually your story, but perhaps it sounds familiar. This story actually represents thousands of adolescents who have come to me for care. Girls and boys. Volleyball players, gymnasts and runners. Singers, actors and 4-H Club awardees.

While the details vary, the typical story is of a superstar high achiever who gets sidelined with an injury or illness and then is so overcome by fatigue, dizziness, nausea or pain that he or she is unable to resume normal activities. Doctors struggle to find answers and teens are left feeling accused that the problem is "all in their heads." If this is your story, rest assured that it's not "all in your head"!

A perspective on medical problems

Many doctors and lots of their patients often focus on identifying "structural" problems — where testing can reveal the specific anatomic structure that is broken, damaged, inflamed or infected. Once the structural problem is found, the solution becomes clear — fix the altered structure.

But more than a third of medical visits relate to specific symptoms for which there are no identifiable structural problems. It's helpful to think of these as "functional" problems, problems for which the structures are fine but the various body parts aren't communicating well with each other. Some functional problems are well known, like the chronic pain of a migraine headache, for example, or the upset stomach of irritable bowel syndrome.

Many of my patients like device analogies that help them understand these two types of medical problems. Structural problems are like the hardware, or actual physical components, of a computer or a smartphone. Functional problems are like the software or the "apps" that run on the computer or phone. When an app doesn't work like it should, it's usually because of a glitch in the networking system or the algorithms aren't "talking" to each other like they should. In a similar way, functional medical problems relate to alterations in communication or networking between body parts due to the nervous system not working well.

A matter of function, not structure

To understand how your body parts "talk" to each other, it helps to know some basic stuff about your nervous system. There are three main parts of the nervous system — the sensory nervous system to feel, the motor nervous system to move, and the involuntary (autonomic) nervous system to regulate blood flow, intestinal flow, and temperature.

Patients with chronic fatigue often have no identifiable problem with a specific body structure. Rather, they have problems of function because the nervous system isn't doing its job properly. When people feel bad with pain (the sensory nervous system not working properly), moving (the motor nervous system being altered), or fatigue with or without dizziness and nausea (the autonomic nervous system not appropriately regulating involuntary activities), there might be a functional disorder rather than a specific anatomic structural problem. We'll talk lots more about the nervous system in the next chapter, but do you already see where this perspective is leading us? This view of the nervous system should be very relevant to everyone reading this book.

Many of my patients come to me frustrated because they or their doctors limited their evaluation and treatment to identifiable structural problems and forgot about the possibility of functional disorders. Finding no evidence of a structural problem and no abnormal test results, they wrongly assume that there is no problem or that the problem exists only in the patient's imagination. We can avoid this by recognizing the reality of functional disorders — in particular, disorders of the autonomic nervous system. In the next chapter, I'll explain the autonomic nervous system in greater detail.

👤 LAURA

"She's just depressed." "There doesn't seem to be anything medically wrong with her." "She just needs to push through." "I don't know what else we can do."

My parents and I kept hearing similar stories from doctors. At first, the doctors were not so skeptical. However, as the plethora of tests they ran on me kept coming back as normal, the doctors' belief in my symptoms seemed to wane. I just wanted someone to listen to me. I wasn't crazy. Something was wrong, and I desperately wanted answers. As the weeks and months passed by with me spending the majority of my time in bed, I questioned whether we would ever find an answer to my declining function.

🧑 LAURA'S PARENTS

At one point during Laura's journey toward a diagnosis her physician called and asked me (Mom) to attend our scheduled appointment without my daughter. Fear set in immediately but I had an inkling about where this conversation might be headed and I was right. As all the numerous and various test results had come back normal the doctor felt it was quite possible that this illness was in "Laura's head." We had quite simply looked at every avenue and the next logical step was to look at depression as the root cause. In fairness, we loved this physician. She was kind, gentle in her approach, and had spent a lot of time with us. This conversation also happened prior to some of the more physical symptoms becoming significant.

As a parent I was devastated because in my gut I knew this was not depression. I knew that my energetic, happy-go-lucky, loving daughter did not just flip a switch one day and become depressed. I will never forget how I felt at this meeting and I will always remember my direct response. I told the doctor that I accepted that my daughter was depressed. Who wouldn't be?

Laura was unable to get out of bed and participate in life. She felt like her wonderful teenage years were slipping by. Instead she was a distant observer of everyone else living a full and exciting life while she sat on the sidelines. Laura spent most of her days alone thinking about all that she was missing. Her once faithful friends were busy with school, work, dating, and extracurricular activities. She could follow their lives through Facebook. She was not with her friends; she was at home with her parents. Social media was a double-edged sword. She was able to stay somewhat connected; however, Facebook was a continual reminder of the life she was missing.

My response to the doctor was this: "I accept that depression is a part of the diagnosis but it is secondary to a primary diagnosis we haven't yet discovered." I understood why the doctor was heading in the direction of such a diagnosis. She had performed every test possible and nothing was showing up, so the next logical step was to look at our daughter's mental health. When I asked the doctor what she would do if this was happening to her daughter, her response was "keep looking" and that is exactly what we did.

My final comment to the doctor was this, "I wish you knew my daughter and the life she led before this illness happened." I think what I was trying to say, was "please listen." "Don't give up on us." This is when she said that she was out of ideas and recommended that we head to Mayo Clinic. As much as you want a diagnosis you quickly realize how much you appreciate a doctor who says, "I don't know what is wrong with your daughter, but I will help you navigate the next step."

One day, early on, Laura was at school when one of her dear friends informed her that she and her mom had Googled Laura's symptoms and they kept coming up with a diagnosis of "just depression." I remember how angry Laura was; it is one thing for the medical profession to expand its search for a possible diagnosis but when people close to you are not validating your illness, it is heartbreaking.

Chapter 4: The autonomic nervous system

Usually, our bodies function without us thinking about them. We breathe in and out regularly. Our blood flows to all the right tissues and organs. Our immune systems identify and repair damaged cells. Our digestive systems absorb nutrients from our meals. All of this automatic activity is controlled by our autonomic nervous systems.

Scientists know a lot about how the autonomic nervous system works. Learning from scientists, you and I can start to understand this part of our bodily function. We can decide if problems in autonomic control might relate to chronic fatigue and if they even relate to you.

One of my sons once forgot to take his trumpet to school. I quietly stepped in to the back of his seventh grade science class to deliver the instrument. Turning to leave, I heard his teacher explaining the roles of T-cells and B-cells. I was astounded. The seventh graders were learning things about medical science that had hardly been discovered when I was in medical school!

So even though many adolescents have already learned things that are more advanced than the medical science I learned, I think it still helps to review basic facts together. We'll get to T-cells and B-cells later, but let's look at the nervous system now.

The nervous system

There are different ways to classify the nervous system. Some people divide it into the central nervous system (brain and spinal cord) and the peripheral nervous system (the nerves that extend from the central nervous system to other parts of the body). In this classification, the autonomic nervous system is considered part of the peripheral nervous system since it runs in chains alongside the spinal cord and from there branches out to other body parts. Of course, though, all parts of the nervous system interact, so there are connections between the brain and the autonomic nerves. Within the central nervous system, the brainstem and hypothalamus regulate some of the autonomic function.

Another way to try to understand the nervous system is to divide it into motor, sensory, and autonomic parts. The motor part does things like make your body move. The sensory part helps you feel things like pain, for instance. And you already know a little about the autonomic part — it guides your body's involuntary functions. All of these nerves and systems interact.

The autonomic nervous system

The autonomic nervous system is made up of nerves that control (regulate) the involuntary or automatic stuff that we don't usually have to think about. Without any of our willful voluntary effort, our bodies seem to know how to make blood flow appropriately to all parts of the body, whether headed "uphill" against gravity toward the brain, for example, or simply running down to the legs. Our internal temperature is regulated to remain right around 98.6 degrees F. Our pupils know how much to open up to allow light in. Our intestines know how to move meals through as digestion happens. Pupil dilation, blood flow, intestinal flow, temperature control — these activities all happen automatically under the control of the autonomic nervous system.

While these body actions are indeed involuntary, we can obviously choose to do some things that impact these functions — like holding our breath to temporarily stop breathing or putting on a jacket to help with temperature control.

Like other nerves, autonomic nerves are long and skinny. They send messages to and receive messages from the distant (peripheral) parts of the body — such as the eyes, heart, blood vessels, intestines, and skin — and regulate these messages in "relay stations" along the spine.

Nerves link across tiny spaces called synapses to other nerves and to muscles. The nerves communicate across these spaces by secreting a variety of chemical messengers called neurotransmitters. The type and quantity of neurotransmitters in the synapse determine what the nearby nerves or muscles will do.

Sympathetic and parasympathetic nerves

There are two sub-groups of autonomic nerves that use neurotransmitters in complementary or, sometimes, competing fashion. Sympathetic nerves generally communicate about quick action needs, while parasympathetic nerves use their neurotransmitters to give instruction to other nerves and to muscles about how to help stabilize and maintain regular body functions. Sympathetic nerves stimulate fast action to respond to danger — like the old "fight or flight" reflex — by increasing output from the heart and decreasing intestinal function. Parasympathetic nerves stimulate rebuilding functions like digestion and intestinal activity.

Sympathetic and parasympathetic functions overlap and interact. The same neurotransmitter chemicals can work on both systems, but the nerves in the different systems balance and interpret the neurotransmitters differently.

Epinephrine (adrenaline) and norepinephrine (noradrenaline) frequently stimulate the sympathetic nervous system. Serotonin is known by many people as a brain neurotransmitter that helps to regulate mood; it's also very active in parasympathetic nerve communication around the intestines as it regulates food flow through the lower digestive system.

Different nerve cells also cluster and work in different patterns. Named for Greek letters, alpha and beta nerve cell receptors receive input designed to stimulate autonomic action. Alpha receptor activity usually increases blood flow and can increase blood pressure. Beta receptor activity usually increases heart rate and opens blood vessels.

This is all pretty cool yet pretty complicated. And it's hard to measure neurotransmitters in action. We can measure levels of some neurotransmitters in blood and urine samples. But these one-time measurements don't always reflect what is going on in real time — in the connecting spaces (synapses) between one nerve and another and between nerves and muscles.

To get a better picture of what's going on, we instead often evaluate patients by seeing how their sweat responses and blood flow react to stimulation, either of the nerves directly or by changing the body's environment.

What does all of this have to do with you?

How does the autonomic nervous system relate to being tired all of the time?

Say communication between the autonomic nervous system and the brain isn't working as it should. This causes poor blood flow, which leads to insufficient amounts of oxygen and other nutrients being delivered to the rest of the body. Lack of oxygen and nutrients causes fatigue. In addition, if blood vessels aren't getting the message to tighten up when you stand, then gravity will pull lots of blood downward with little resistance from floppy blood vessel walls, leaving you dizzy from a lack of blood flow to the head. Similarly, if the intestines don't get proper autonomic input, they may over-contract (painfully) or under-work (nauseatingly so). It's at least plausible that some of your problems might relate to poor autonomic control of blood and intestinal flow. Fatigue, dizziness, and nausea can, indeed, result from dysfunction of the autonomic nervous system.

👤 LAURA

I just finished my first year of medical school, and if I could summarize what I learned into one sentence it would be this: The human body is extremely fascinating and incredibly complicated. The way I see it, and drawing upon my love of music, the functioning of the autonomic system is like an orchestra. The conductor is the main regulator — the sympathetic and parasympathetic nervous systems — telling the musicians what to do. The conductor knows when a crescendo or grand pause is needed throughout the symphony and signals for the musicians to do so — just like the sympathetic nervous system should tell your blood vessels to constrict when you stand up to make sure blood isn't pooling in your hands and feet. The musicians, on the other hand, are tasked with carrying out the conductor's vision. I like to think of them as the individual's nerves, neurotransmitters, and synapses. They get told what to do by the conductor and then need to perform. Unfortunately, my body's orchestra seemed to be out of sync. Maybe it just needed a little more rehearsal time.

——— ————————————————————————————————————

Chapter 5: Mitochondria, muscles, and marathons

Some readers might feel like they've already got all they need from this book. They feel sleepy-tired, and they now have ideas about how to improve their sleep duration and quality. They also understand how their involuntary nervous systems regulate normal activity.

Most chronically tired adolescents, however, don't simply feel sleepy-tired. They also feel blah-tired. They're tired, but they can't recover just by sleeping. Sure, better sleep would be part of the solution, but they need more than just more sleep. Often, it's even hard to get to sleep. These people lack energy.

To begin to understand how to overcome this kind of fatigue, we need to learn a bit more about how the body works. We need to know about two energy machines in the body. We'll get down to the microscopic level and consider very small energy producers — the energy factories that live in each cell of the body. These little microscopic energy machines are called mitochondria. Next, we'll need to look at the big picture with energy users — the body's muscles. We'll need to consider how the muscles turn chemicals into action. We'll see how muscles get work done.

Many tired people are tired because their bodies have become inefficient with energy production and use. When we understand how mitochondria and muscles work, we'll be able to understand how to deal with fatigue and even overcome some of our fatigue.

Microscopic energy factories

Early in medical school, I learned about the Krebs cycle. The Krebs cycle is a series of chemical reactions that take place in tiny structures inside our cells called mitochondria. The Krebs cycle takes oxygen along with sugar, fat, and protein to produce energy. This energy comes in little chemical packets called adenosine triphosphate (ATP).

The Krebs cycle is like an app that's always on in the background but to which we pay little attention. We breathe in air and about 21% of that air is oxygen to power the Krebs cycle. We eat food, which is basically a combination of sugar, fat, and protein — even though it comes in all sorts of forms and tastes. These are the essential ingredients for energy production. Inside our cells' mitochondria scattered all over our bodies, the air and food combine to produce little ATP packets of energy. These packets are then transported within the body to power the working action of other cellular processes.

Energy production problems Complicated energy production works well when things are in balance. But sometimes this balance gets upset for a variety of reasons.

For example, some people have mitochondrial diseases that block parts of normal ATP production and lead to the buildup of toxic wastes. This can cause strokes, exercise intolerance, and weakness. Mitochondrial diseases are rare. But knowing how these diseases occur makes us wonder if even minor imbalances in mitochondrial function (that are still poorly understood) might lead to more subtle inefficiencies with energy production, such as chronic fatigue.

Genetics also may have an effect on energy production. Some teenagers with chronic fatigue have mothers who also have or have had chronic fatigue. Since the genes controlling mitochondria come only from the mother (without paternal influence), some people have wondered if chronic fatigue can be inherited from mothers. This hasn't been proven yet, and current research makes it doubtful that maternal genes are the only cause of chronic fatigue.

Mitochondria also require iron to support their energy-producing machinery. Interestingly, about half of teenagers and adults with chronic fatigue are low on iron (as measured by testing their ferritin levels). Fatigued adult women get more energy when they take iron. Should all tired teenagers take iron? No. But tired teenagers should see a doctor who can test to make sure that their ferritin level (iron store) is adequate. If it isn't, then iron supplements could be helpful.

In addition, we know that people who don't use sugar normally, such as people with diabetes who are also overweight, can knock their mitochondria out of balance so that fat gets overused to produce energy. This leads to the production of unusual semi-toxic

⏱ QUICK TAKE

Energy to run our bodies is produced in tiny mitochondria in the form of ATP. If we are among those people who have a diagnosable condition that interferes with energy production, then specific treatment might help us get more energy. But what about the average teenager who is tired but doesn't have a mitochondrial disease, iron deficiency, or diabetes? Knowing about these other conditions teaches us that our bodies' energy production is a pretty complex process and that at the very least, it's important to take good care of our mitochondria. We can do this by eating a balanced diet while avoiding too much sugar and too much fat. We should keep our weight within a healthy range — and that's a struggle for at least a third of teenagers these days.

---

forms of oxygen (free radicals) that can hurt other parts of the body and block healing processes.

Muscles, users of energy

A friend of mine is a lung doctor who studies exercise. He has a personalized license plate that reads "VO2 DOC." What's that about?

VO2 refers to the uptake of oxygen into the muscles. It's a number that comes from an exercise test. The test shows how efficient the muscles are at using the oxygen that's in the blood. The "V" stands for the rate of uptake or consumption, and the "O2" refers to oxygen (O_2). The amount of oxygen taken into the cells and used up at full exercise is called the maximum oxygen uptake, or VO_2 max. It basically shows the muscle machine's potential maximum capacity for converting oxygen to action.

VO_2 max is usually measured using a treadmill or a stationary bicycle to let a person exercise while attached to a bunch of tubes and wires. These "cardiopulmonary exercise tests" — similar to the stress tests that older people undergo to see how their hearts tolerate stressful exercise — give lots of information about how a person's pulse,

WHAT ABOUT COENZYME Q10?

Coenzyme Q10 is a substance in the body that facilitates part of the energy-producing Krebs cycle. Research in mice shows that supplemental coenzyme Q10 helps mice swim farther before they get tired. Research in Japan shows that otherwise healthy people can accelerate faster when riding a bicycle if they take coenzyme Q10 supplements. A few adults with chronic fatigue felt a bit better when taking supplements, but we don't yet know if this effect is significant enough to suggest supplements for other tired people. Research into mitochondrial function continues, but we don't yet have enough evidence to suggest coenzyme Q10 supplements for tired teenagers. And my tired patients who tried coenzyme Q10 pills didn't feel any more energy with the pills than without.

blood pressure, and breathing patterns respond to exercise. And these tests show how efficient the muscles are at taking in oxygen. Essentially, the higher a person's VO_2 max, the more efficient his or her body is at using oxygen.

Chris Froome, a recent repeated winner of the Tour de France bicycle race, reportedly has a VO_2 max of 88. Most fit athletes have numbers around 60 or so. Average teenage boys are usually at 45 or higher, and adolescent girls are usually at least 35. There are lots of factors that determine a person's VO_2 max.

Factors affecting muscle oxygen use Genetics seem to affect how a body uses oxygen. Scientists are just beginning to learn about the relevant genes, but there is probably a genetic reason why Kenyans and Ethiopians seem predisposed to use oxygen efficiently enough to keep winning marathons.

Age and gender affect VO_2 max, as well. VO_2 max tends to peak during the late adolescent and early adult years. Males tend to have higher VO_2 max levels than females, regardless of whether they are sedentary or athletic.

By far, though, the greatest impact on VO_2 max comes from conditioning. The more a person exercises, the more efficient at using oxygen (fit) that person gets. This fitness is separate from strong, toned muscles, but it comes similarly from exercise. Aerobic (cardio) exercise conditions the cardiovascular system, leading to aerobic fitness and improved VO_2 max levels.

How exercise can help conquer fatigue What do VO_2 max and conditioning have to do with tired teenagers? Exercise is a key component of treating chronic fatigue. The more we exercise, the greater our VO_2 max and the better we are at producing energy and using it efficiently. To increase VO_2 max, tired teens must condition their muscles with physical exercise to make better use of energy. Often, tired teenagers feel like they have no energy. In a way, they're right. When they undergo exercise tests, they often have VO_2 max levels that measure in the teens and 20s.

These tired teens breathe in oxygen, but the mitochondria in their muscles aren't working efficiently enough to turn the oxygen into ATP (those little packets of energy we discussed on page 64) to get them moving and doing things. Their minds might be motivated and they might try hard. But their muscles, big or small, are inefficient.

This sort of conditioning takes time. It's kind of like learning to play a piano or to type on a keyboard. The more we do these activities, the smoother, quicker, and more natural our movements become. It's the same inside our muscles. The more we push our muscles to make increased use of oxygen by exercising, the more efficient our cellular mechanisms become to get that oxygen cycling through the Krebs cycle and coming out as ATP.

On the other hand, physical inactivity quickly leads to deconditioning. We know from studies of patients placed in intensive care units that lying in bed with little movement can lead to deconditioning and shrinking of the muscles in a matter of days. Muscles quickly lose their efficiency at using oxygen. (This is made even worse if the person has to use a steroid medicine like prednisone while inactive.)

⏱ QUICK TAKE

One of the paradoxes of chronic fatigue is that people feel too tired to exercise, but the treatment for chronic fatigue is to exercise. Exercise will increase VO_2 max levels, which will improve energy use. The key is taking that first step.

For example, say you want to learn how to type so you can use your computer keyboard efficiently. You have to learn how to place your fingers and practice moving them in the right directions to get fast at typing. Similarly, tired teenagers need to put their bodies in motion (even when they don't feel up to it) and then practice doing it every day. Over time, they can gradually increase physical activity as tolerated so that their bodies become more efficient at using oxygen.

I sometimes ask patients who've had chronic fatigue and gotten better to explain the key to their recovery. A common response is "Exercise, exercise, exercise."

Exercise did not even seem in the realm of possibility when I first became sick. I could barely make it through a class period without falling asleep, so when one of my doctors suggested that I try to exercise throughout the week, the thought was laughable. Luckily, I started to work with a personal trainer at my gym who encouraged me to get moving, even though I could not work out like I had when I was swimming competitively. We started slow — with walking and Pilates. At first, it really did not make me feel any better. It was incredibly difficult to fight through my symptoms and drag myself to the gym, knowing that I would not automatically see results.

Marathon lessons

It's often said that recovering from a chronic illness is like running a marathon, not a sprint. Indeed, many people are helped by taking a long-term, marathon-like approach to recovery. For me, I've also learned a lot about my tired patients and their condition by running.

Whether you've been an athlete or not, there are likely some lessons for you in reading about what I've learned from running, lessons that can be valuable, as they relate to conquering fatigue and economizing energy.

Lesson 1: Don't skip the basics I started running during college. Initially, it was for a mental break from studying. I would run around the hills and cow pastures that surrounded my campus. I got more serious about running in medical school, mostly because my mind was so loaded that I needed even more mental breaks. I ran in a few short races and then entered a full 26.2-mile marathon.

This was during the 1970s. There was a then-new idea about carbohydrate loading to help people run long races. The idea was to starve one's self of carbohydrates for a few days and then to "carbohydrate load" the night before the race. (The idea lives on, at least in the spaghetti dinners served before some major marathons.) So for one particular marathon, I stopped eating carbohydrates the Tuesday before the Saturday race; I ate lots of protein. I got busy Friday evening, though, and forgot to do the key carbohydrate loading part of the plan. From the first steps of Saturday's big run, my legs felt heavy and my mind felt sluggish. I battled on for 21 miles and then quit.

Can tired teenagers seeking recovery learn anything from my aborted marathon? I hope so.

No matter how long one prepares and no matter how hard one tries, bodies get worn out if we neglect the basics. My poor mitochondria were starved, starved in a good way that increased their efficiency. But then I left them starved when they needed the carbohydrates to support my running legs. My failed marathon yielded a future message: "Don't skip the basics." Anyone trying to recover from fatigue must give attention to the basics, such as a balanced diet and regular sleep.

Lesson 2: Learn to focus your energy By understanding factors that determine how fast elite runners can cover 26.2 miles, we can all learn things to help us achieve our own maximum potentials, especially if we're dealing with significant fatigue.

The efficiency of oxygen uptake (VO_2) is clearly a factor in marathon success. But, another factor rivals VO_2 as a predictor of success — running economy. Running economy is a measure of oxygen consumption while running at a given pace. Basically, it is the VO_2

per distance covered. Some people are less "economical" runners because their body movements include extra energy-consuming activities that don't promote forward progress. They might flail their arms or bound higher with each forward step.

How is "running economy" relevant to tired teenagers? It reminds us to work within our limits. We're not built to run 70 miles per hour like a cheetah. But if the goal is to cover a certain distance — or complete a specific academic or social task — we will be more likely to have success if we improve the "economy" of our activity.

Out for a leisurely jog one time, I was headed east as the sun was setting. I watched my shadow and noticed that I waddled a bit from side to side. I realized that I was wasting lateral energy that could have been directed forward. It was as if I was sending my little ATP energy packets into the ditch beside me instead of using them to run forward. I modified my running style and was able to run faster with less effort.

Whether someone is an elite marathoner, an aging pediatrician, or a tired teen, we all can learn to focus our energy forward in line with the priorities of what we want to accomplish. And we can work to avoid wasting energy on lateral, nonessential tasks.

What do I mean by this? People with chronic fatigue aren't as good at multitasking as other people who don't have chronic fatigue. If we realize this, we will focus on one task at a time, and we will try to do things in order rather than all at the same time. We will remove distractions that slow our forward progress.

For instance, fatigued patients in research studies do better at academic tasks if they don't have distracting sounds in the background (even pleasant music can be distracting). Our success in accomplishing a goal — our "task economy" — goes down when our minds (or bodies) keep wandering in other directions or bounding higher in directions we're not intended to go. The marathon analogy teaches us to FOCOS:

- **F**igure out what our goal is
- **O**rient our minds directly toward that goal
- **C**oncentrate on the targeted outcome
- **O**vercome distractions (even good, fun distractions that consume our energy without advancing us toward our goal)
- **S**avor the pleasure of victory as we successfully complete tasks

Marathon science, it seems, can teach tired teenagers to 1) exercise to improve VO$_2$ max and 2) maximize activity economy by focusing on the task directly at hand. Multitasking is inefficient!

Lesson 3: Adjust expectations At the same time, though, marathon science reminds us that some things may be beyond our control. Genetics, for example, have some influence on success in running and other sports. One gene relates to angiotensin and oxygen use and is associated with marathon success in Spanish runners but not in Kenyan runners. Another gene related to a chemical called actinin is associated with success in power sports but not in endurance running.

Even while we're still learning more about genetic factors related to enduring through fatigue, we do know that we are all unique and that our bodies have different abilities. That goes for marathon runners as well as tired teens. A clear lesson for chronically tired teens is that we should adjust our expectations rather than thinking we can excel at everything all the time.

Other things we can control. Only rarely do elite marathon runners weigh more than 160 pounds. Their muscles are toned, and they carry very little unnecessary fat. We want whatever energy we do have to go toward useful activity, not just carrying around extra weight. Heavy shoes can slow marathon runners. Heavy bodies can slow tired teenagers. We all need to keep our weight appropriate for our height.

Lesson 4: Turn negatives into positives Another factor related to running economy is the ability of the muscles to absorb energy during the mechanical shock of landing and then transfer it to the pushoff of the next step. Again, this provides a great analogy for dealing with fatigue.

Since my running is mostly motivated by a desire for mental breaks, I particularly enjoy running in new areas, especially scenic or stimulating areas. Landing at Reagan National Airport one August evening, I got a ride to a hotel and laced up my shoes. An hour later, I was headed for "the Mall" in Washington, DC — not the shopping mall but the park-like walkways lined by government buildings and museums. Unfortunately, my body was accustomed to comfortable Minnesota weather. The 98-degree temperature and 98% humidity hit me hard. Half a mile into my run, I felt totally drained. My legs were heavy, and my mind sagged. I felt totally nonenergetic — just like the patients I had seen earlier that week with chronic fatigue.

Even small steps in normal weather sometimes leave my patients feeling drained, heavy, and unable to continue. But, it was the example of a particular young woman with fatigue that kept me going on this hot August evening. Realizing and even feeling somewhat how she felt and knowing that she kept up with her college classes despite her fatigue, I kept moving. Up around the pool by the Capitol and then back down to the Lincoln Memorial, I jogged. Mentally, I used my bad physical feelings as a reminder of a successful patient. This kept me motivated to move forward. It turned out to be a great run, even though I felt exhausted through most of it. I realized how even everyday activities can feel like marathons for many of my patients.

Marathoners need to absorb the "trauma" of the foot hitting the pavement. They need to store up this energy in a way that helps their leg muscles spring back to push the foot upward again. Physically and mentally, tired people need to absorb their bad feelings and use them to propel themselves forward.

A running friend of mine grew up in the highlands of Kenya and ran six miles to and from grade school each day. To some of us, this seems pretty near impossible. But my friend's accomplishment was due to the fact that every day he rose to the challenges he met. Exposure to high altitude challenges our ability to use oxygen efficiently. But continuous exposure gives our muscles experience dealing with low oxygen supply, which helps build our maximal oxygen uptake. Exercising, as we talked about before, also challenges our ability to use oxygen. Exercising regularly helps build that efficiency. Combining both challenges of high altitude and exercise additively increased my friend's VO_2 max, allowing him to run with ease in the mountain air. The natural tendency of tired teenagers is to lie around, but that makes our VO_2 max drop and it makes subsequent exercise even harder. Instead, we can train ourselves to see the challenge of fatigue as a reason to build activity into our daily lives.

Lesson 5: Put all the pieces together Decades after my failed marathon attempt, I entered another marathon. The weather was perfect — a sunny but cool day along the shore of Lake Superior. It was 2004 and my 49th birthday. Each step of the run seemed to bring lessons for dealing with fatigue. First, mental stuff matters. The motivating music of the *Chariots of Fire* theme song blared from loudspeakers at the starting line and stuck in my mind for miles. Second, we are not alone. Thousands of other people were conquering their past failures and current fatigue to join in the race. Two friends, in better shape than I was, ran the first seven miles with me. Their conversation inspired me and encouraged me. Third, preparation is important. I had run miles and miles for months before the race and probably had my VO_2 max higher than ever before in my life; this made the first 19 miles of the marathon incredibly enjoyable. I loved it! Fourth, the basics always matter. I had enjoyed a macaroni feast the evening before the race and felt ready. My muscles were getting the carbohydrate supply they needed. Fifth, the basics still matter. I thought it was pretty nice that I wasn't sweating on the cool sunny day. Too late, I realized that I should have been sweating. I hadn't been keeping up on fluids during the early miles of the race. I was drying up. My legs cramped. My mind faltered. We all need to drink enough fluids, especially when dealing with fatigue (be it chronic or exercise-induced). Finally, we're still not alone. My wife and kids were at mile 22 to cheer me on. They kept me going even when I felt like quitting.

Winning your marathon

Tired teenagers have plenty of reasons to be frustrated by their limits as they see peers passing them by, but we all have limits. Whether patients or elite athletes, we can all strive to maximize our mitochondria, move our muscles, and master our own marathon experiences — whether those experiences involve sports or just getting through a morning at school.

⊞ NOTES FROM A NURSE

Most of the teens I work with are highly motivated and tend to be perfectionists … so they share a lot with the typical distance runner! Because of this, however, I know if I push them they will try whatever I tell them to do … at least once. So if I say "To get better, you need to go out and run five miles!" most of them would go out and try this. Some might actually succeed in that they finish this distance. However, they would then "crash," feel horrible, and it would take them days to recover. The lesson they then learn is "Exercise makes me feel horrible!" Not at all the goal! Whether you are training for a marathon or working up to 30 minutes of daily aerobic exercise, you need to start off slowly and work your way up. No successful marathoner waits until race day to run more than a 5k. Start off with a shorter distance, and work your way up to the race (and recovery).

Distance runners often talk about "hitting the wall" — reaching that point in the race where, for whatever reason, you suddenly feel that there is no happiness left on the Earth. That your legs cannot move another muscle, and that you are going to die if you don't quit running. Hitting the wall can be demoralizing, and it is easy at that point to quit: to give up, stumble off the course, and go home.

In POTS recovery, ups and downs are also common. Too often, our patients start off in kind of a "honeymoon" phase, where things are going well, they are feeling great and it's pretty easy to buy into the recommendations of salt, fluids, and activity. Then comes an illness, a seasonal change, a stressful event (either physically or emotionally). Suddenly, their symptoms flare and they find themselves struggling. It's easy to get discouraged, believe that all of their hard work is for nothing, and that they will never feel better again. They have hit the wall.

Runners are told to focus on the basics when this happens. Have a drink, eat a snack, pull on a phrase (such as "I am strong!") to keep going and redirect focus. When teens with POTS hit the wall, they also need to focus on the basics. Hone back in on what you have been doing for your salt. Look at your fluids. Dial back (but don't completely quit) your exercise. Know that this is just a setback. It is not the end. The race is still on. This is not the finish.

— Jeannie, who has run marathons

Chapter 6: Lessons from history

Before we move ahead, let's go back a few years in history. Let's see how doctors began to link autonomic dysfunction with chronic fatigue and all these other symptoms. We'll consider first what space travelers have been learning about fatigue and dizziness since the 1960s, review what autonomic specialists discovered in the 1990s, and then see what doctors more recently started learning from their patients with chronic fatigue.

Space cases

People with poorly functioning autonomic nervous systems often find it hard to think clearly. They have trouble concentrating. Occasionally, they're accused of being "space cases." Perhaps there is hidden wisdom in the accusation!

While studying history, my children once asked what monumental things had happened in my lifetime. I put "A man walked on the moon" near the top of my list. My children were flabbergasted and exclaimed, "You were alive that long ago?"

Yes. I was in high school when Neil Armstrong took his "giant leap" for mankind. I watched television footage (in black and white!) of astronauts returning from space. But they weren't celebrating their victories with fist pumps or energetic dances in the end zone. Instead, these astronauts were so weak that they had to be helped out of their space capsules and lifted onto stretchers to be taken for medical care.

What was going on with these "space cases"?

Spending days without the influence of gravity, astronauts' bodies adjust. Their blood flows smoothly throughout their bodies, and their autonomic nervous systems make the muscles around blood vessels settle into a state of relaxation. When they return to Earth, however, their autonomic systems aren't quite ready. It takes hours to days for their bodies to relearn how to make blood flow against gravity. Until they readjust to being on Earth, astronauts can feel overwhelming fatigue, dizziness when upright, and even nausea.

I know. You haven't been to space. But if you experience both fatigue and upright dizziness, maybe your body has somehow "forgotten" to adjust to changes in position; maybe the automatic part of your nervous system has forgotten how to deal with gravity. When upright, maybe you can no longer keep blood flowing appropriately. You're not a mental "space case," but perhaps your body is acting a bit as if it is in space. You, like the astronauts, have "orthostatic intolerance"— an inability to adapt to, or intolerance of, the change in position from lying down to standing upright.

Advancing medical science

During America's Civil War (and again during the world wars of the last century), many soldiers were unable to continue military service due to what was called irritable heart or soldier's heart. (This is not to be confused with a distinctly different but concurrently described form of Civil War syndrome, which was psychological in origin and featured fear and anxiety.) Soldiers with irritable heart had fatigue, dizziness, palpitations, headache, chest pain, and disturbed sleep. For many of them, careful questioning revealed that their trouble had started even prior to their entering the military. No specific cause was identified, and heart medications were sometimes given.

Around the same time as the Civil War, a doctor named William W. Mayo got tired of being sick with malaria every summer in Indiana. So he moved to Rochester, Minnesota. He and his wife raised their boys to become doctors, too. Meanwhile, he used a horse and buggy to make house calls for the local population. When a tornado wiped out houses and injured many people, a group of Catholic nuns convinced the good Dr. Mayo to provide hospital services to recovering tornado trauma victims. His sons followed him into practice.

Over the years, the reputation of the hospital and clinic, staffed by the Mayo brothers, grew favorably. People journeyed from far beyond the local farms to seek care from one or another of the Drs. Mayo. Clinic staff grew numerically and led the way at the forefront of medicine. More and more people came with increasingly complex problems that had not been solved by experienced doctors in other areas of the country.

In January 1993, more than a hundred years after Dr. Mayo first moved to Minnesota, Drs. Ronald Schondorf and Phillip Low published a report of several adult Mayo Clinic patients who had excessively fast heart rates when shifted from a lying down (supine) to a standing position. These patients were mostly women and frequently had developed fatigue and dizziness with, often, sluggish intestinal flow following a viral illness. Drs. Schondorf and Low labeled this "idiopathic postural orthostatic tachycardia syndrome" and suggested that it was due to a problem with the autonomic nervous system.

Over the subsequent years, these and other doctor-scientists at Mayo, as well as other interested physicians around the world, identified many other similar patients and further characterized the problem. Frequently, these patients also had abnormalities in the way they sweated in addition to the unusual way they adjusted their heart rates to positional changes.

In 1996, Dr. Low and his colleagues reported on some adolescents who similarly had postural orthostatic tachycardia syndrome, or POTS. In Japan, a 16-year-old boy was identified with POTS in 1999. In 2000, Dr. Blair Grubb in Ohio and Dr. Julian Stewart in New York each detailed more adolescents with POTS. Adolescents were being diagnosed with POTS with such frequency that some wondered if this was a new epidemic. The truth is, people were just becoming more aware of the condition and diagnosing it more often.

In the past decade, careful evaluation of patients with chronic fatigue reveals that many have abnormalities in the function of their autonomic nervous systems. If soldiers in the 1800s had been evaluated, they, too, probably would have shown autonomic abnormalities.

My experience with POTS

Shortly after I came to Mayo Clinic in 1999, I started seeing patients in a pediatric diagnostic and referral clinic. The idea was that I, as a general pediatrician, would see children coming from around the United States who had problems that didn't fit into a specific specialty area of pediatrics. I was quickly overwhelmed with teenagers with chronic fatigue and, often, chronic pain. I saw so many tired teenagers that I wondered what was going on. I thought about calling the pattern of post-infectious fatigue I was seeing the "Hitting the Wall Syndrome"— these were high achievers who seemed to "hit the wall" of a mono-like illness and then wilt. A neurologist friend asked if these patients might have POTS, and I wondered what marijuana had to do with it! My friend explained POTS, which I'll describe to you in detail in the next chapter. I'd never heard of it. So, I started checking my patients' pulses in different positions and found that, indeed, a majority of the tired teenagers did qualify for a diagnosis of POTS.

Sadly, I was not alone in my ignorance at the start of the new millennium. Even today, many physicians still haven't heard of POTS. Many teenagers remain undiagnosed and miss out on helpful treatment.

Connecting the dots

But before we describe more about what POTS actually is and what we can do about it, let's go back in history again. Let's see what we've been learning about chronic fatigue and how affected individuals often have dysfunctional autonomic nervous systems.

In the mid-1990s, a uniform definition of chronic fatigue syndrome was proposed. This was designed to help researchers better compare patients, treatments, and outcomes. Otherwise, as chronically tired patients know, there are often well-meaning people suggesting things like, "My aunt's cousin's neighbor was just like you. She took (whatever) treatment and is fine now. You should try that."

Chronic fatigue in general means people are tired for a long time. But chronic fatigue syndrome is defined as meeting three criteria: 1) severe fatigue for more than six months that isn't related to any identifiable medical diagnosis or test, 2) fatigue that interferes with daily activities, and 3) the presence of at least four of these eight specific symptoms:

- 24 hours or more of tiredness after physical exertion
- Unrefreshing sleep

- Impairment of short-term memory or concentration
- Muscle pain
- Multiple joint pains without swelling or redness
- New sorts of headaches
- Frequent or recurring sore throat
- Tender swollen lymph nodes in the neck or armpits

Of course, there are lots of other medical conditions that can cause these symptoms, so it's important that people don't get labeled as having chronic fatigue syndrome without first identifying and treating any other conditions that might be present.

In the late 1990s, some doctors in New York were working with teenagers with chronic fatigue syndrome. The doctors decided to test the teens' autonomic nervous systems. One of the most important tests of the autonomic nervous system is to see how the flow of blood changes when the person is held upright. Doctors call this the "head up tilt" test. A person lies down while supported on a special table. The table then gently tilts so it's nearly upright (usually angled at about 70 degrees). The person is still and supported so as not to require any use of leg muscles. This allows doctors to test the person's heart rate (pulse) and blood pressure while working against gravity and without using the big muscles of the arms and legs. This test shows how the autonomic nervous system, separate from the skeletal muscles and voluntary effort, regulates blood flow.

Among the teenagers with chronic fatigue syndrome, almost all (25 out of 26) felt terrible when tilted; 18 had racing hearts; and seven fainted. This provided clear evidence that at least some people with chronic fatigue actually have poorly functioning autonomic nervous systems. The researchers also found that people with chronic fatigue syndrome have unusually static (unchanging) heart rates when resting and that they lack some of the normal variations of up-and-down changes in pulse. This is similar to what happens in people with POTS. This all suggests that the sympathetic and parasympathetic parts of the autonomic nervous system (see page 57) aren't appropriately balanced.

A few years later, a research group in Norway showed that when upright, teens with chronic fatigue have stronger sympathetic responses than parasympathetic responses. The group also found that teens with chronic fatigue sweat differently than normal teenagers and that the abnormal sweating was related to changes in neurotransmitter (catecholamine) responsiveness. In 2011, the Norwegian researchers reported that they had found a variation in the genetic makeup of the beta neurotransmitter receptors in people who had chronic fatigue syndrome.

Clearly, the autonomic nervous system is out of equilibrium in many people with chronic fatigue syndrome.

ⓥ QUICK TAKE

So where is all of this leading? We have good clues from history. War history tells us that symptoms of chronic fatigue and dizziness have been around for a while and that these symptoms can keep young people from performing vital activities. Space travel history shows us that it doesn't take long for a body to "forget" how to deal with gravity. International medical history shows us that many chronically tired people have abnormalities in the way their autonomic nervous systems control blood flow and sweating. These historical themes have converged at Mayo Clinic into a greater understanding of postural orthostatic tachycardia syndrome (POTS).

Now, with all that background, let's get on with it. Let's see what this POTS stuff is all about and what we can do to actually get better.

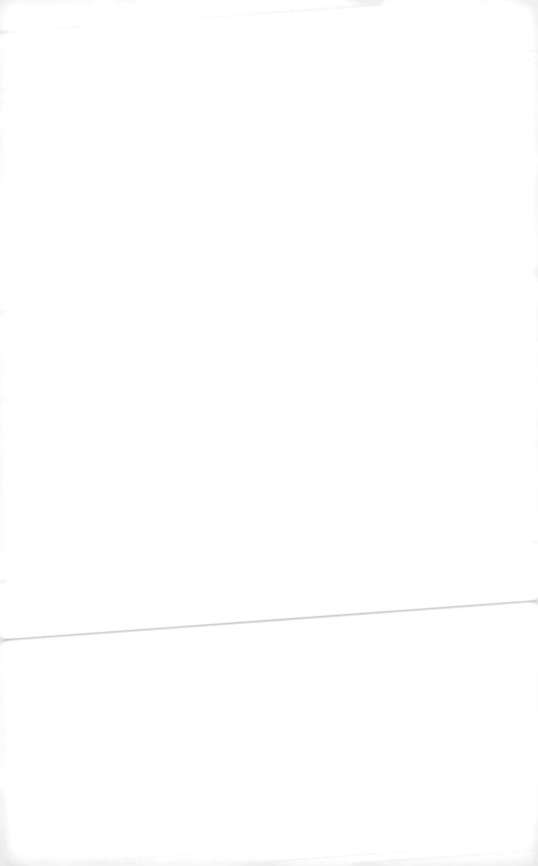

Section 3: What is POTS?

Chapter 7: POTS!

Now if you've been reading the whole book up to this point, you understand that feeling tired is common among teenagers. Often what's needed for many of these teens is simply to slow down their schedules so that they can get to bed on time and get quality sleep.

But you also learned that there are lots of other causes for fatigue in teens, such as lack of iron, anemia, or problems with hormones, kidneys, liver, or the digestive system. Some tired teens have a readily identifiable medical problem that improves with treatment. This is why it's important for teens to see their doctors when they feel tired all of the time and don't know why.

A chronic feeling of fatigue and lack of energy could also be a problem with your autonomic nervous system and how it communicates with the rest of your body. Many teens who have chronic fatigue may boost their energy level by making basic lifestyle changes like getting enough rest, eating a variety of nutritious foods, maintaining a healthy weight, and getting plenty of exercise.

But there's another group of tired teens whose fatigue is part of a complex condition known commonly as POTS. We're now going to turn our attention to that particular problem.

Defining POTS

POTS stands for postural orthostatic tachycardia syndrome. The terms *postural* and *orthostatic* in postural orthostatic tachycardia syndrome are used a bit redundantly, but the words combine to refer to changing position (postural) so as to be upright (ortho) and still (static). Normally, when a person is postural and orthostatic, the heart rate sometimes goes up a bit for a brief moment.

For someone with POTS, the heart (cardia) beats unusually fast (tachy). This is known by the term *tachycardia.* And all of this is associated with symptoms — dizziness with postural changes, fatigue lots of the time — that add up to make a syndrome.

In plain language, POTS is a condition of bothersome symptoms associated with excessive increases in pulse when the body's position changes from lying down to upright. But what is POTS to the person experiencing it?

If you're a teenager with POTS, it can be a miserably frustrating condition. You're tired all of the time but struggle to sleep. You get dizzy when you stand up, and your brain seems foggy. It's hard to remember things and to concentrate. You feel nauseated a lot, and you have pains. POTS is miserable.

If you love someone with POTS, you feel bad, too. You see your child or friend wasting away. He or she looks normal but just can't do much. You try to be encouraging, but you feel like a nag. You back off and see your loved one dwindling more. You want to help but have no clue what to do. You're frustrated and you want to find answers.

If you're a doctor, you realize that POTS is still relatively unknown but is much better understood than before. And you are probably seeing patients with fatigue and dizziness who likely have this condition.

👤 LAURA

POTS can be terrible. There's really no way to sugarcoat it. Symptoms can come and go sporadically, so it's kind of like waking up every day as a game-show contestant. "Let's see what's behind Door Number 2! Congratulations, you just won a day of nausea, dizziness, and headaches!"

My mind and my body weren't on the same page. I so desperately wanted to participate in life, but my body just wouldn't cooperate. For me, POTS felt like living in a body that was working against me.

👥 LAURA'S PARENTS

Defining POTS is difficult, as it is a condition that is always in flux. The best way to describe it is that you are going along with your normal happy life and one day someone comes along and pulls the rug out from under you and you are left with a life you do not recognize.

Or pretend you are a major character in a video racing game. You are in last place on a course you do not know, and all the while you are trying to get to the finish line, roadblocks are popping up with no rhyme or reason, setting you further and further behind simply because they can. No one ever tells you where the finish line is or when it will come

Or here is another analogy. Your body has been taken over by a 3-year-old who wants to do what he wants, when he wants, without warning. Over time you forget what normal is and have absolutely no knowledge of how to get back on track.

✚ NOTES FROM A NURSE

The typical patient that I see in the clinic is a white adolescent girl. She is smart, high-achieving and usually either an accomplished student or an athlete (or both). She tends to also be the kind of girl that people just "like" or are drawn to. Life for her has usually seemed to be going pretty well, when all of a sudden she gets an illness, she gets an injury, she wakes up wrong one day and WHAM. All of a sudden she and her family find themselves playing a game of medical whack-a-mole as they desperately try to manage one symptom while others keep popping up. This girl is not lazy; she is not crazy. Something wrong is going on.

— Jeannie

A closer look

Let's dig a bit deeper into the medical definition of POTS. We want to understand this condition well.

A critical component of a POTS diagnosis is a rapid increase in heart rate when standing up. In POTS, this unusually fast heart rate is tied to a chain of events that link back to the autonomic nervous system (remember Chapter 4?). When a person with POTS stands up, the autonomic nervous system isn't doing a good job of telling blood vessels in the legs to tighten up and send blood flowing back to the heart. Instead, the vessels stay floppy and the blood pools in the legs. As a result, the heart tries to make up for inadequate blood flow by pumping faster, increasing the heart rate.

Measuring this increase and making sure it's due to the autonomic nervous system, and not other factors, can be a little tricky. To rule out other causes of accelerated heart rate, it's important to be truly still when upright. But this is hard to do. You're not a skeleton or a statue. Most people tend to move around a bit and to shift their positions. All of this uses muscles. When muscles contract, they squeeze on nearby blood vessels and make them contract to push blood onward. So your muscles can sometimes make up for autonomic nervous system failures.

How hard is it for the average person to stand completely still? You can test this out in a living room or medical office. A living room is more comfortable, while being in a medical office might make some people nervous, which might make their pulse rate higher than normal. Wherever you are, you should lie down still and comfortably rest for several minutes so your circulatory system adjusts. You can then check your pulse (the number of times your heart beats in a minute). Then stand up totally still (or as close to still as you can manage) for a few minutes and have someone recheck your pulse.

How long? Standing for just 30 seconds or a minute doesn't allow enough time for your body go through all of the normal adjustments to position. Stand for too many minutes and some might faint — and give up on a career as a guard at the Buckingham Palace.

Usually, three to five minutes is a reasonable time to stand still. Of course, even this might be hard for someone with POTS who subconsciously knows it is healthier and safer to wiggle around and shift positions to help the blood flow.

The head-up tilt test

It can be difficult to get an accurate result at home, though, because most of us can't stand perfectly still. We fidget and sway. Then, when someone is trying to find our pulse, we interact and might even laugh or complain that their fingers are cold on our wrists. All this can make the pulse go up for reasons that are totally separate from POTS.

So we doctors try to remove some of this variability. We check the pulse while the person is lying down facing upwards (supine) on a special tilt table. Once the resting pulse has stabilized, the table tilts up. The person is held comfortably on the table with straps, so he or she doesn't need to use muscles to support the upright position. Because the straps would be too uncomfortable if the person was totally upright, we usually tilt people at about a 70-degree angle. Using this head-up tilt test, we can standardize the environment (tilting 70 degrees for five to 10 minutes) and find the difference between the supine and standing heart rates.

How much of a heart rate difference between the two positions is normal? In the early 1990s, doctors evaluated a group of adults and found that people with the symptoms of POTS had pulse changes of more than 30 beats per minute; healthy people with no symptoms have lesser pulse changes. This 30-beat-per-minute change was appropriately accepted as the criteria for a diagnosis of POTS.

Making room for variations Seeing tired teens, however, my colleagues and I noticed lots of variation in pulse changes. Seeing healthy teens for checkups and other minor medical issues, we started checking pulse changes in people who weren't suspected of having POTS.

(One of my sons even did a high school science fair project on this topic. He checked supine and standing heart rates in 26 friends. One of his healthiest subjects, a cross country runner at the peak of fitness, had a pulse change of about 40 when changing from lying down to being upright.)

My colleagues and I then went into a couple of our local high schools and checked about 300 sophomores. We did some statistical analysis with their pulse changes and found that even seemingly healthy adolescents can have pulse changes of up to 42 beats per minute. Subsequently, we took about 100 teenagers into the autonomic laboratory and did head-up tilt tests on them. Again, the statistical analysis shows that healthy adolescents can have pulse changes of up to about 40 beats per minute with tilting and that teenagers with POTS have greater changes in pulse.

So we now use a 40-beat-per-minute change in pulse as the cutoff level to differentiate teenagers with POTS from people without POTS. Of course, we must be careful not to be overly rigid. "Normal" pulse changes do not shift dramatically on the day a person stops being a teenager. And a person's symptoms are probably more important to the diagnosis than the details of his or her pulse change. Some people seem to have POTS even though their pulse doesn't change much with tilting. The actual diagnosis of POTS requires both symptoms and excessive pulse change.

The role of blood pressure Initially, adults couldn't be diagnosed with POTS if they also experienced a drop in blood pressure with standing. A decrease in blood pressure when standing upright is a different condition called orthostatic hypotension. People with orthostatic hypotension might faint, but they usually don't have chronic fatigue. What about teenagers? It seems that tired adolescents are spread over a spectrum of pulse and blood pressure changes. Indeed, some do have big changes in pulse and marked drops in blood pressure.

Though doctors still debate exact definitions, most agree that POTS implies an excessive increase in heart rate separate from any drop in blood pressure. Of course, for some people with POTS, blood pressure does fall and they even faint after they've been upright with an excessively rapid heart rate for a while. Abnormal regulation of heart rate and abnormal regulation of blood pressure are varied manifestations of similar problems in the autonomic nervous system.

Getting the whole story

It's important to remember that POTS is a clinical diagnosis. That means a diagnosis of POTS doesn't rely on test results alone, but also on other factors, including symptoms and medical history. A medical professional who is familiar with POTS should make the diagnosis after carefully considering the patient's whole story and test results.

There are other medical problems that have excessive heart rate upon standing as a symptom but which are distinct from POTS. Or these same conditions can overlap with POTS. These other conditions include:

Dehydration and blood loss Dehydration (as seen with severe vomiting and diarrhea with inadequate fluid intake) and blood loss (like after an auto accident with a ruptured spleen) lower the volume of circulating blood. Whenever the blood volume drops, the body compensates by increasing the heart rate, especially when upright. When symptoms are sudden and short term, postural tachycardia usually indicates the presence of low blood volume (hypovolemia).

Anxiety and pain Anxiety and pain also elevate the pulse. Sometimes, anxiety and pain increase with postural changes and make it look like there is a primary autonomic problem when the autonomic system is actually just adjusting to an outpouring of anxiety- and pain-related neurotransmitters.

Deconditioning Deconditioning also increases the degree of postural tachycardia. Deconditioning, as experienced by astronauts in our earlier example, can relate both to cardiac function and to muscle function. The inefficiency of cellular energy metabolism can be the underlying cause. So, astronauts returning to Earth's gravity have excessive postural tachycardia, but they don't have the clinical story that goes along with a true diagnosis of POTS. People with POTS have long-term (chronic) intolerance of an upright position, in addition to other symptoms.

All of this is a bit abstract and theoretical. Let's personalize things a bit in the next chapter and further consider the symptoms of POTS. What does POTS actually feel like?

Chapter 8: Symptoms, symptoms, and more symptoms

Having a medical label such as POTS gives doctors a shorthand way to talk about groups of patients. And accurate labels help researchers compare different groups of people in a meaningful way. But that doesn't change the fact that each person with POTS is unique. Each person with POTS experiences his or her own particular set of symptoms.

We also realize that tired, dizzy patients share a lot of symptoms regardless of whether or not their heart rate changes when they stand up. So some medical labels are broader than others. For example, we say teenagers have autonomic dysfunction or orthostatic intolerance if they experience fatigue and dizziness without an excessive heart rate change. We say they have POTS, which is a form of autonomic dysfunction and orthostatic intolerance, if those same symptoms are associated with an excessive increase in pulse when upright.

In this chapter, I explain both common and uncommon manifestations of POTS, and I talk about some related conditions that may overlap with POTS.

POTS IN CONTEXT

People aren't born with POTS. POTS happens. It comes on suddenly in some people, especially after an illness or injury when they're laid up and temporarily inactive. In others, the symptoms start and build up much more gradually over several months. POTS can occasionally occur on top of other medical concerns (like stomachaches since kindergarten), but it usually happens in previously healthy people.

What are some of the factors that people with POTS have in common? Many of them are adolescent girls or young women — about two-thirds of adolescents with POTS are female. In addition, POTS is diagnosed primarily among Caucasian and Asian people.

Most adolescents with POTS start to experience symptoms around the time their bodies are going into puberty. Some, though, develop POTS during later adolescence, and there are adults (90% of whom are women) who get POTS during their middle-age years.

Statistically, POTS is most common in high achievers. There seems to be a link between being highly motivated with great successes in life and then getting POTS.

So the "average" adolescent with POTS is a previously high-achieving girl who started having trouble when she was about 12 years old. There is a wide range, though, around this average patient.

There are lots of similarities among people with POTS, but not everything is the same. We must be careful not to overgeneralize the situation.

Fatigue

Fatigue is the theme of this book, and fatigue is the core of POTS. It is the unifying feature common to most all POTS patients.

There are two main forms of fatigue — sleepiness and simple lack of energy. Some people have both. Some feel sleepy but then can't fall asleep. Most people with POTS, though, tell me that they aren't particularly sleepy; they simply don't have energy. They don't feel up to doing much at all.

The tiredness of POTS is sometimes worse when standing upright. Rarely, patients will say that they feel fine when they are lying down; it is only when they stand up that they feel drained of energy. Most of my POTS patients, though, are tired all of the time. They might feel a bit more tired when they are vertical, but they're tired almost all of the time.

Though we don't understand why, many people with POTS are especially tired in the morning. Their energy levels start perking up a bit at around 10 or 11 a.m., allowing them to feel less tired, but still not letting them feel normal. This makes attendance at morning classes particularly difficult.

👤 LAURA

At the height of my symptoms, the worst part of POTS was the extreme, unrelenting fatigue. No matter what I did, or how much I slept, the fatigue did not wane. I was always so perplexed. How can I sleep for 20 hours and not feel even the least bit refreshed? I had a variety of other symptoms as well — headaches, nausea, brain fog, dizziness, tachycardia, sweating, and noise and light sensitivity. It wasn't just the physical symptoms, though — I also felt extremely isolated. My friends were amazing, but they just couldn't understand what I was going through. Everyone else was sitting in math class talking about [the homecoming dance], and I was wondering if I would feel well enough to make it through the rest of the school day.

The fatigue of POTS can wax and wane over time. It's usually less severe when schedules are lighter — summer vacation, for instance. It tends to get worse with increased levels of activity, which is why our patients tend to feel especially bad when school starts back up in September each year.

Sleep deprivation makes the fatigue worse. Teenagers with POTS are particularly worn out when they become ill, such as when they get colds. Menstrual periods may seem to make all POTS symptoms, including fatigue, worse.

People with POTS typically have post-exertional fatigue. After an unusually strenuous activity, they feel more tired than usual, even a day or so later. Unfortunately, it is this after-exercise fatigue that convinces some people with POTS to not even attempt to exercise. (The better option in this case is to start out with a light exercise regimen and gradually increase the intensity and frequency of the exercises, as you'll see later in the book.)

Why are people with POTS so tired? With POTS, the involuntary nervous system doesn't regulate blood flow properly. The circulatory system doesn't get the right amount of blood to the right place at the right time. Undersupplied with oxygen and nutrients, the body can't keep up with the demands placed on it and grows tired. So inadequate blood flow seems to be the basis of tiredness in people with POTS.

At the same time, though, POTS is linked to faulty neurotransmitter levels. If you'll recall, neurotransmitters are the chemical messengers that carry signals from one nerve to another. Decreases in some neurotransmitters (or imbalances between the various neurotransmitters) can give a perception of fatigue in addition to the tangible tiredness of undersupplied body parts. This is not just an "in your head" perception of tiredness but a true physical tiredness arising from nerve synapses scattered all over the body.

Dizziness

Almost all people with POTS feel dizzy, but they describe the feeling in different ways. For me, dizziness and lightheadedness are the same thing. The head feels airy and perhaps even floating. As dizziness worsens, thinking becomes difficult. You feel wobbly. Shadows appear around the edges of wherever you're looking, and vision can narrow down to a central tunnel. All vision can be lost and, of course, extreme dizziness leads to fainting.

Talking to a 15-year-old with POTS, I asked if she was dizzy. She said, "No." I asked if she was lightheaded, and she again said, "No." Surprised, I kept listening for hints of dizziness and heard none. Later, I asked how her eyes were. "Fine," she replied," except when I am blind." Startled, I asked when she was blind. "Every time I stand up," she explained, "I go blind for 15 or 20 seconds." I still don't know if she had the blindness of severe dizziness without the sensation of dizziness or if she was so accustomed to feeling dizzy that she didn't recognize those feelings as abnormal and worthy of mention.

Medically speaking, dizziness is different from vertigo. Vertigo is a sense of the room spinning around you, rather than feeling unstable within the environment. True vertigo comes from problems of the inner ear rather than from the altered blood flow that occurs with

PADDLING A CANOE TO COMPREHEND POTS

Why is dizziness a symptom of POTS? That's relatively easy to explain. Our blood vessels are surrounded by small smooth muscles. These muscles are stimulated or relaxed by neurotransmitters from autonomic nerves. Tightening of the muscles narrows blood vessels. Relaxation of blood vessels opens them wider. With POTS, the autonomic nervous system is out of balance in a way that tends to leave the blood vessels wider than usual — more floppy, with decreased smooth muscle tone.

I like relaxing canoe rides in southern Minnesota. Floating gently downstream for hours, I have watched bald eagles soaring overhead, and I have seen deer bound across the river. I was even chased by a group of angry geese. My adult children sometimes go with me, but they actually prefer the more rapidly moving rivers with whitewater and more energetic thrills.

What's canoeing got to do with POTS? Well, when a river is wide, the water flows slowly and gently. As the river narrows, the water rushes through more rapidly. In the same way, wide-open blood vessels allow the blood to slow during its circulatory course, and tighter blood vessels speed the circulating blood on its way.

With POTS, blood tends to pool in floppy, poorly contracted blood vessels in the lower parts of the body rather than circulate as it should. As a result, less blood continues its upward course, and less blood than usual reaches the brain. The heart tries to compensate by beating faster — trying to send blood out to the body more frequently. Still, not enough blood gets to the head, and the person with POTS feels dizzy.

POTS. But for unexplained reasons, some people with POTS experience both dizziness and vertigo.

Sick to my stomach

People with POTS commonly experience nausea and abdominal discomfort.

Just as blood flow is regulated by tightening and relaxation of tiny muscles around blood vessels, so food is propelled through the intestines by gentle involuntary squeezes of muscles that are wrapped around and along the intestines. These intestinal (enteric) muscles are controlled by autonomic nerves. The mechanisms are the same as for blood circulation, but the enteric nerves are part of the parasympathetic nervous system (see page 57) rather than the sympathetic nervous system that controls circulation.

When blood vessel muscles undertighten (or overrelax), blood pools in the lower parts of the body and people get dizzy. So when stomach and intestinal muscles undertighten, you might expect the digesting food to stagnate, producing a feeling of nausea, the sensation that the stomach is too full and needs to empty itself by vomiting.

That makes sense, and it's partly true. But we did a little research to see if this is really the full explanation or not. We looked back at a few dozen teenagers who seemed to have POTS and who also had problems with nausea. To learn more about their nausea, we tested the rate at which their stomachs emptied (gastric emptying). We had them eat some eggs containing a small, safe amount of radioactive substance and then measured how quickly the stomach pushed the radioactivity further down into the intestines. About a fourth of the patients had very slow stomach emptying — which was what we expected. But half of the patients had normal gastric emptying, and the remaining fourth were rapid emptiers.

What does that mean? It means the problem is one of irregular control of flow. It's not that intestinal flow is always too slow or too fast. It's that the flow through and beyond the stomach varies too much. Sometimes it's too fast, and sometimes it's too slow. Normal body function requires smooth changes and transitions depending on what the person is doing (standing, lying, resting, running, eating or using the toilet). The abdominal problem with POTS is that intestinal flow isn't always appropriate to the circumstances.

During times when gastric emptying is too slow, people with POTS probably feel nauseated. During times when the intestines are trying to move things through too quickly, spasms and crampy pains may occur. It's a bit like Goldilocks — sometimes things are too fast, sometimes things are too slow, but they never seem "just right."

Some people with nausea feel better when they eat; others feel more nauseated after eating. Some have frequent abdominal pains but feel better after passing stool; others feel worse in the bathroom. The issue is that people with POTS have poor control of intestinal flow. This results in nausea and pain at various times in various people.

Headache

About 60% of the adolescents who see me for symptoms suggestive of POTS have bothersome headaches. Many have constant headaches that vary in intensity but never go away. Most feel pain in the front and sides of their heads, and they describe the pain as explosive or pressure-like.

Sometimes the headaches are associated with worsened nausea or even vomiting. Only occasionally do my patients have the typical tension headaches in the upper neck and at the back of the head.

If the blood flow in my head changed erratically, I'd probably have a headache, too. For people with POTS, though, it's not clear whether the headache is mostly a side effect of altered blood flow or of other changes in central nervous system neurotransmitters. It's interesting that beta blockers help prevent migraines in susceptible people (even without POTS), and beta blockers also help treat blood flow problems in people with POTS. In any case, POTS and headaches often do get tangled up together. Whatever the physiology, headaches usually improve as POTS gets better.

People with migraine headaches are often bothered by bright lights. Sometimes, people with POTS also are bothered by light; this can be because the pupils over-dilate and allow extra light to enter the eyes.

If you have POTS, it's important not to ignore your headaches. Don't assume that all headaches are just a part of POTS. If a headache is unusually severe or wakes you up at night, you need to seek urgent medical attention. As it is with anyone else, such a headache may be a sign of a problem unrelated to POTS, such as a brain tumor.

Pain

Teenagers with POTS often have lots of other pains. This isn't surprising since the neurotransmitters that are associated with POTS are the same as or similar to the neurotransmitters that communicate pain to the brain.

Some people with POTS develop chronic pain at the site of a previous injury — such as a back, arm or leg injury. Others develop back pain, perhaps related to a lack of normal physical movements and activities.

As with headaches, though, we shouldn't assume that all pain experienced by people with POTS is happening because of POTS. I have a POTS patient who struggled with abdominal pain — until a surgeon removed his inflamed appendix, a problem that needed its own separate treatment and had little to do with POTS.

Usually, pain serves a purpose. It warns us that something is wrong and that we should take action — whether pulling a foot out of a hot bath or getting a broken arm set and casted. Sometimes, though, the sensory nerves "get confused" and keep repeating pain messages — even when there is no danger and when no urgent action is required. Confused autonomic nerves and confused sensory nerves seem to hang out together!

Chest pain in people with POTS sometimes seems related to changes in blood flow between the chest and the abdomen. This may be associated with shortness of breath and a sense of not being able to breathe. For some, this seems like a panic attack — except that there was no panic prior to the chest pain and troubled breathing. I think that these brief "POTS attacks" are probably due to a combination of altered blood flow in the chest and altered nerve sensation. Fortunately, these brief episodes of chest pain aren't dangerous.

Symptoms of fibromyalgia and POTS overlap a lot. Fibromyalgia refers to chronic pain that centers mostly in the muscles, and it's often associated with fatigue and poor sleep. In fact, POTS is likely the underlying cause of what seems to be fibromyalgia in some adolescents. The peculiarity of fibromyalgia is that it's also associated with tenderness in some parts of the muscles. Treatments for POTS encompass essentially all of the treatments for fibromyalgia, so a person with POTS doesn't need to do anything different just because she or he also qualifies for a diagnosis of fibromyalgia.

It's helpful to rule out treatable causes of pain so that they can be treated appropriately. Once these are taken care of, it is easier for a person with POTS to understand the difference between acute pain that points to a separate problem and chronic pain. For chronic pain, appropriate pain management strategies can be instituted even when no specific cause is found. This prevents wasting time and expense looking for the cause of unexplained pain and allows improved focus on successful recovery.

Brain fog

One of the most frustrating symptoms of POTS is that thinking seems to get clouded. Patients have told me it feels like their "brain is in cobwebs" or that their "brain is covered with cotton candy." Many call it "brain fog" since their thoughts feel foggy or cloudy. They have to slow down to search for words and ideas just as drivers in the fog need to slow down to look for traffic and road markings. In a sense, dizziness is the physical feeling of a sluggish mind, while brain fog is the mental feeling of slowness of thought.

Many people with POTS-induced brain fog feel like they can't remember things. They report staring at friends whose names they are trying to remember. Or they forget where they put their keys. Interestingly, on actual memory testing, people with POTS do fine. Neuropsychological testing usually shows that people with POTS have good memories and excellent cognitive (thinking and planning) skills.

Why then do my POTS patients feel like they can't think when testing shows that they actually can? It might be a matter of focus. On neuropsychological testing, the person is totally concentrating on the test, with no distractions. In real-life situations, the need to recall names and details comes amidst a loud, distracting world with lots of other demands on multitasking teens. For people with POTS, their minds can work well, but they also get overwhelmed and don't work as well in real-world settings where multitasking is required.

That can't be the whole explanation, however, because many people with POTS feel mentally sluggish even when they're not in distracting settings. While some brain fog can be overcome with effort and exertion to think, another part of brain fog is probably due to the brain being undersupplied with what it needs to think. What does the brain need to think? It needs oxygen and nutrition, including salts and all the right chemical details. When blood flow is compromised — as it always is with POTS, especially when upright — brain cells are undersupplied with the fuel they need to function properly. What else does the brain need to think? It needs neurotransmitters, those chemicals that serve as messengers of thoughts and actions. People with POTS have altered levels of the neurotransmitters required for smooth blood flow, and they likely have altered levels of the "thinking" neurotransmitters.

So brain fog is a challenge. It likely results from the POTS-affected brain's struggles with multitasking, the lack of steady blood flow, and alterations in neurotransmitter levels. Medical science hasn't yet advanced to the point of knowing exactly how to restore neurotransmitter balance. We treat adolescents with POTS as best as we can, but brain fog and sleep difficulty seem to be two of the last symptoms to resolve as people recover from POTS.

Blue feet

It's fairly normal for blood to pool in the lower legs of people with POTS when they're upright. As the blood stagnates, it doesn't get replenished with oxygen. The feet and ankles can swell and turn bluish. Blood flow slows. Skin, stretched by the swelling of pooled blood, can feel tingly or even painful. Moving around can quickly improve blood flow and get the feet (or hands) back to normal color.

One of my colleagues likes to tentatively diagnose POTS by greeting his patients with handshakes. When a chronic fatigue patient has cold hands, he thinks POTS is likely. When he sees the lower legs swelling and turning blue when the patient is standing still (waiting for the pulse to increase) he is further convinced that part of the problem is POTS-induced pooling of the blood.

Raynaud's phenomenon is a condition where cold temperatures cause the hands or feet to change color and become uncomfortable.

This can be similar to the blue feet of POTS but usually isn't position dependent and usually involves red or white color changes rather than bluishness. A few people with Raynaud's phenomenon also have lupus erythematosus, a chronic inflammatory disease that can be debilitating. Correctly diagnosing the blue feet or hands as part of POTS can relieve concerns that other conditions, such as Raynaud's or lupus, may be causing the person's symptoms.

Palpitations

Increased activity (and increased stress, for that matter) can make the heart beat faster and harder than usual. Sometimes, the heart even feels like it's pounding through the chest. Anyone can feel these "palpitations," but people with POTS are more prone to these sensations than others, especially right after they stand up and start to feel dizzy. They feel like the heart is suddenly working faster than normal because the heart is suddenly working extra hard to make up for the blood that is uselessly pooled in the legs.

With POTS, though, the heart should beat regularly, even if it is beating fast and hard. If the palpitations feel like skipped or irregular heartbeats, then it's worth getting checked out by a doctor. Usually, though, even skipped beats aren't dangerous in adolescents. Increased use of caffeine and other stimulants also can aggravate palpitations.

Hot stuff

One of the key tasks of the autonomic nervous system is to regulate the body's internal temperature. When POTS affects the circulatory, gastrointestinal and sensory nervous systems, it can also interfere with the autonomic control of temperature (thermoregulation).

Some people with POTS feel too hot, and some feel too cold. One of my POTS patients wore shorts during winter even though she lived in the snowy Rocky Mountains. Another wore thick sweatpants in the middle of a hot, humid Texas summer. Too hot or too cold — people with POTS often don't feel like their temperatures are right.

The average human body temperature usually varies between about 97 and 100 degrees F. With POTS, the temperature varies a lot within this range and sometimes goes a bit outside of this normal range. Somehow the nerves "automatically" controlling temperature aren't able to smoothly regulate body heat.

On the other hand, it's pretty rare for a person with POTS to have high fevers unless there's an infection or some other problem. Some parents and teens I know have spent way too much time measuring, recording, and graphing temperatures. We already know that POTS affects temperature control, and the exact numbers don't usually change the diagnosis or lead to other helpful treatments.

Some of the newer thermometers that measure skin temperature will seem to vary even more. Since blood flow throughout the body is abnormal, blood flow to the skin also is irregular. When there's less blood going to the skin, the surface temperature (as measured by some thermometers) is low. When blood flow increases, the temperature registers artificially high.

When people are cold, they involuntarily shiver. The muscle contractions of shivering generate heat to warm the body. When people are hot, they sweat. Sweating leads to evaporation, which cools the body. As temperature control varies in people with POTS, they sometimes feel shivering chills. At other times, they sweat excessively. Some adolescents with POTS even "sweat the bed." Their pajamas get so wet that they need to get up to change clothes during the night.

Thinking outside of POTS

POTS explains lots of symptoms, but it doesn't explain everything that bothers each of my patients. Not every symptom someone with POTS has is due to POTS. Similarly, not every other condition a person with POTS has is related to POTS. This is the same in the rest of life, too. For instance, just because someone has blond hair and POTS, we can't believe that the hair color caused the POTS or that the POTS caused the hair color. Everyone has more than one defining characteristic, and not all of those characteristics are directly related to one another.

I have seen patients with POTS who also had inflammatory bowel disease, celiac disease, autoimmune hepatitis, and cancer. None of those conditions, though, are any more common in people with POTS than in the general population. The occurrence of two serious conditions in the same patient seems simply coincidental in these situations. Some conditions do seem to be more common in people with POTS. But on closer inspection, the connection isn't always there.

Asthma When we reviewed a few hundred of our POTS patients, we found that about 30% had been diagnosed with asthma. This is about twice as high as in the regular population. With detailed questioning and testing, however, we found that many of our patients didn't actually have asthma. It seems that their POTS attacks combined with exercise intolerance prompted other doctors to incorrectly suspect asthma. In fact, asthma and POTS don't seem to be linked in any more than random fashion.

ADHD Some conditions seem less common in people with POTS. For instance, attention-deficit/hyperactivity disorder (ADHD) is found in about 11% of children overall. But in the last three thousand patients I've seen with POTS, the incidence of ADHD seems much, much lower than that (only about 0.1%). The neurotransmitter abnormalities of ADHD likely move in the opposite direction of the neurotransmitter imbalances of POTS, so it's unusual for someone to have both conditions.

Chiari malformation Chiari malformation is a condition where the back of the brain sags lower than usual and crowds the spinal cord as it exits the base of the skull.

Most Chiari malformations are mild downward displacements at the edge of the opening in the skull that don't cause any clinical symptoms or pose any danger. But for some people, the sagging brain compresses the spinal cord to the point of causing headaches and neurological problems.

Some people suggest that Chiari malformations can cause POTS, and we've seen a few teenagers with both problems. It's important to make sure the Chiari malformation is severe enough to really cause the symptoms, however. The operation to repair a Chiari malformation involves opening up the skull and moving the brain around. We wouldn't want to perform such aggressive treatments unless we knew the malformation was really the issue.

Hypermobility A majority of adolescents with POTS have very flexible bodies. This helps for sports like volleyball and gymnastics. When the body's soft tissues are loose, though, there is less rigid support around blood vessels. This means that when blood vessels fail even a little to contract, there can be more trouble with floppy blood vessels, pooling of blood in the legs, and POTS.

There are several genetic conditions, such as Ehlers-Danlos syndrome, that make bodies extra flexible. Whether or not someone with POTS has an identifiable form of Ehlers-Danlos syndrome (and some, but not all, forms can be identified with genetic testing) doesn't change the diagnosis, treatment, or outlook for POTS.

So even though Ehlers-Danlos syndrome is fascinating, I rarely do diagnostic testing for it. I focus instead on treating the POTS and on treating the joint laxity with physical therapy. It's important for people with hypermobility to do exercises to strengthen the muscles around the joints on a regular basis.

Spells Prolonged fainting. Seizures. Spells. Some people with POTS have prolonged episodes where they seem to lose consciousness. Typical fainting episodes last only a few seconds and resolve when the head is placed level to the heart. Spells in some people with POTS can last for several minutes or even an hour or so. Sometimes these episodes are associated with awareness that comes and goes, and with unusual seizure-like body movements.

Of course, several dangerous conditions can manifest as episodic spells of abnormal consciousness and muscle activity. So people who experience spells may need to undergo testing to rule out heart rhythm problems and actual seizures.

Sometimes, we'll hook patients up to wires that measure brain waves (electroencephalogram or EEG) and monitor their brain waves during spells. Often, we'll get an electrocardiogram (EKG or ECG) to see what the heart is doing in general and, sometimes, during spells as well. If these tests are normal, then we can lower our worry level and accept the episodes as non-dangerous spells.

So, what causes these spells in patients with POTS? Most likely, there's a disconnect between the impulses flooding the peripheral nervous system and the overwhelmed brain. Regular life can be overwhelming as it is for teenagers. But POTS is constantly overtaxing the nervous system with abnormal, "confused" neurotransmitter messages. Wherever the subconscious brain is, it gets overwhelmed trying to regulate conflicting nerve messages. With autonomic and sensory input bombarding the brain with sometimes inaccurate and inappropriate messages, the subconscious transforms or converts the messages into a call for a "timeout." Just like the basketball player who yells for timeout when trying to gain more time as the clock ticks down, sometimes the nervous system of a person with POTS takes a break — a timeout — by turning off normal function. Interestingly, these neurological timeouts usually look like fainting (even though tests show conscious activity in the brain), seizures (with jerky movements or overtight muscles), paralysis (usually of an arm or a leg or two), or blindness. The person is not "faking it" or consciously trying to trick people. Rather, the subconscious mind (not open to conscious thought) is transforming the cacophony of overwhelming nerve messages into a timeout.

Spells like this aren't limited to people with POTS who have chronic abnormalities in nerve stimulation levels. Psychiatrists know that similar spells can occur in people who have acute (short-term) stresses, like watching a terrible accident or being assaulted. In those situations, the acutely overwhelmed mind also can take a timeout. Psychiatrists call these episodes a "conversion disorder." This is probably somewhat similar to what happens with POTS. Sometimes, psychological techniques and — when there happen to be physical warnings of spells — physical therapy techniques can help a person deal with POTS-related spells.

Anxiety and depression As mentioned before, POTS is not a condition that's all in your head. But the same neurotransmitters that are messed up by POTS also relate to a person's mood and to problems such as anxiety and depression.

In a sense, anxiety is the opposite of apathy. Apathy is the lack of caring and motivation. Anxiety is a heightened state of motivation. So anxiety is good, to a degree. It is anxiety that keeps us motivated to study before a test. It is anxiety that helps us focus during sports events and pull out a final surge of adrenaline-charged effort. Anxiety can be helpful.

But too much uncontrolled anxiety can be unhealthy. Anxiety leads to the production of more stomach acid to help quickly digest food to prepare for a big physical effort (whether fight against danger or flight from danger). Excessive stomach acid without subsequent physical activity, though, leaves the stomach acid burning through the stomach lining, leading to painful gastritis and ulcers. In addition, too much anxious worry about a test prevents some people from focusing on the things they need to study.

I've seen many people with POTS who have a tendency toward anxiety. They are the high achievers who have excelled in life — until POTS set in and slowed everything down. They still are highly motivated to figure out their disease and to get back into action. I applaud their motivation and, yes, even their anxiety.

But anxiety must be managed. Motivation without action can be self-destructive. So people with POTS need to channel their motivation (anxiety) into positive, productive directions. When their anxiety is getting out of control, they can benefit from talking to a mental health specialist and, sometimes, from taking anti-anxiety medication.

We used to think that depression (rather than apathy) was the opposite of anxiety. But lots of people suffer from both depression and anxiety at the same time. Just like neurotransmitters messed up by POTS can cause too much and too little blood flow in different parts of the same person at the same time, so too can they cause some people to have their mood going in both anxious and depressed directions at the same time.

Sure, some people may have been depressed or anxious before they developed POTS. Treatment for each condition can help. I'm a bit surprised, though, that not all people with POTS are depressed. Having a body that refuses to do what it should can be discouraging and depressing. If we knew what neurotransmitter balance keeps some people with POTS positive and forward looking and motivated for recovery, we would bottle those neurotransmitters to share them with other people. (Or, better yet, we'd find out what specific neurotransmitter balance prevents POTS in the first place.)

As POTS symptoms get better, POTS-induced discouragement (and depression) also can improve. At the same time, though, people with POTS should get all the help they need — including treatment for anxiety or depression. Just because someone gets anxiety or depression on top of POTS doesn't imply that POTS symptoms are psychological or less real.

Gotta go Rarely, people with POTS have so much disruption of their underlying autonomic nervous systems that their toileting habits get way out of balance. This can affect either the urinary or the stool system.

Of all the POTS patients I've seen, only a few (certainly less than 2%) have had trouble with urine output. Some feel like they always have to go and can't. Others go frequently. Since urinary problems are rare with POTS, they require prompt evaluation for other underlying causes. But if indeed it is the POTS causing the urine troubles, then special medication (like pyridostigmine) can sometimes help.

Constipation can be an issue for anyone. But for some people, stool habits vary as their neurotransmitters vary. In a few patients, we see severe constipation with pelvic floor dysfunction in association with POTS. Gradually, the muscles at the base of the pelvis get stronger and stronger. They end up overcontracting. Eventually, when it is time for those muscles to relax to allow the passage of stool into the toilet, the muscles tighten instead of relaxing. This leads to terribly painful constipation. In addition to receiving POTS treatment, these patients often benefit from physical therapy maneuvers designed to retrain the muscles of the pelvis.

Symptoms – so what?

We've reviewed lots of different symptoms and conditions that go along with POTS. But wait! Keep in mind that this isn't a contest. You should not be keeping score to see how many symptoms you have. You don't necessarily have better or worse POTS based on how many symptoms you have or based on how many parts of your body are affected. Rather, each person with POTS has a collection of symptoms, his or her own personalized syndrome. By understanding the symptoms, we should be better able to leave the symptoms behind and move toward recovery.

First, though, some of you still want to know: Why do these symptoms occur? The "what" and "how" of symptoms is not enough for you. So the next chapter reviews more of the "why," what we know (and, unfortunately, don't yet know) about the causes of POTS.

Chapter 9:
Causes of POTS

So, what causes POTS in the first place? We don't truly know. As scientific inquiry continues, though, we can discuss some of the potential causes and triggers of POTS.

Genetic factors

Is a gene responsible for the development of POTS in adolescents? If so, knowing about it would sure help medical scientists predict (and maybe prevent) the development of symptoms. And, if we could figure out what proteins are generated by a "POTS gene," we might then be able to come up with better treatments.

Some diseases come from a specific gene mutation. Sickle cell disease, for instance, results when part of the beta globin gene on the 11th chromosome is altered. (People generally have 23 pairs of chromosomes; the 23rd pair includes a pairing of X and X or X and Y chromosomes related to sex.) This alteration makes red blood cells fragile and results in life-threatening anemia. In the U.S., the gene is most common in Black people and is found least often in white people.

Other diseases have more-complex causes. Diabetes is more common in some families than others. So is obesity. There are genes that relate to these conditions, but it takes more than a single gene abnormality to cause either diabetes or obesity. We call these conditions"multifactorial"since there are many different factors — genetic and environmental — that contribute to their development.

What about POTS? POTS has been diagnosed primarily in white teens, although it's been seen in adolescents of other racial and ethnic backgrounds. And quite a few adolescents with POTS have a parent or sibling who had similar symptoms in their teen or young adult years. These features suggest that there may be a genetic component to POTS, at least in some people, but it's likely not the whole story.

Family history Most doctors ask about family members' health when evaluating patients. My experience indicates that about 15% of adolescents with POTS have a close family member who struggles or struggled with chronic fatigue or dizziness. Perhaps this is due to a gene being shared between relatives. Or perhaps some families are exposed to either physical environments or behaviors that make POTS more likely. A group of Dutch researchers evaluated adolescent girls with chronic fatigue and found similarities in symptoms and health between the affected girls and their mothers (but not their fathers). One explanation for this could be that the "fatigue gene"is located in the mitochondria and, therefore, is inherited only from mothers.

Interestingly, though, in the Dutch study, the more hours the mothers worked outside the home, the less fatigued the adolescents were. Perhaps the issue is less due to genes and more due to psychological or behavioral influences of being around a tired mother. Those researchers suggested that"the shared symptom complex of mother and child is the result of an interplay between genetic vulnerability and environmental factors."

Catecholamine genes Catecholamines are nerve impulse transmitters like epinephrine (adrenaline) and norepinephrine that are involved with blood flow.

A very rare condition related to catecholamines is called dopamine beta-hydroxylase deficiency. In that condition, a mutation on the 9th chromosome prevents affected people from making an enzyme that breaks down the dopamine chemical into norepinephrine. I've only seen two people with it. The lack of this enzyme causes severe orthostatic intolerance that typically starts during infancy and then worsens in adolescence and adulthood.

The parents of one girl with this condition told me they thought she was just a clumsy child, because she kept falling over when she was learning to walk. They later realized that she had been falling over because she was so overwhelmingly dizzy.

Dopamine beta-hydroxylase deficiency can look a bit like POTS. But there are only about a dozen people with this condition in the world, and it doesn't explain most cases of POTS.

Researchers in Tennessee have studied norepinephrine transporter genes and a few other genes. Mutations in some of these genes are found in a few people with POTS, but these genes don't seem to be responsible for POTS in very many people. A series of genes was tested in adults with POTS in Minnesota. None of the genes was related to the risk of getting POTS, but some genetic variations involving catecholamine receptors and transporters were related to how much the heart rate rose in patients with POTS who were upright.

It's complicated So I do suspect that POTS is partly genetic in origin. It seems unlikely that there is a specific single gene *causing* POTS, though. Maybe POTS is genetically more like diabetes and less like sickle cell disease. Perhaps there are multiple genes that predispose a person to getting POTS, but we haven't found many yet that relate to very many people.

Most likely, there are several genetic factors that combine to alter a person's risk of getting POTS, and then there are other genetic risk factors that influence the way a person responds to POTS. As a wise person once said, "It's complicated." While science keeps marching on, we also need to explore other factors that might cause POTS.

Infection

Certainly, people get tired when they have infections. Some infections, like mononucleosis due to Epstein-Barr virus, lead to tiredness that lasts for more than just a few days. I picked up hepatitis A from a patient once (that'll teach me to pay more attention to washing my hands!) and was tired for nearly 10 months. Might chronic fatigue and POTS be due to infection?

Many adolescents with POTS noticed their fatigue and dizziness started while they were sick with an infection or during their recovery period. Often, the initial infection was with the mononucleosis virus or an influenza virus (the H1N1 flu virus was particularly problematic). I've also seen POTS that followed Lyme disease and lots of other North American infections. In Australia, chronic fatigue can follow rickettsial infections. In New Guinea I saw a boy who got POTS after having malaria. And I've seen POTS after brucellosis and schistosomiasis in Africa.

No, you aren't supposed to understand what all of these diseases are! Rather, the point is that POTS often starts with or after an infection, and it doesn't seem to matter much just what the infection is. Minor infections like colds don't usually lead to POTS, but whatever infections lead to more illness and more fever in the local geographical area can be the same infections that lead to POTS in that area.

So, do the infections cause POTS?

In almost all of the people with post-infectious POTS, the infection is long gone by the time POTS is diagnosed. In fact, their bodies have already developed healthy antibodies to prevent them from getting the same infection again. There's no sign that an *active* infection relates to POTS. Rather, it seems like the infection triggered the body to go on to develop POTS, but didn't necessarily cause it.

Might there still be a different hidden infection that smolders along to keep POTS going?

Sure, some people with human immunodeficiency virus (HIV) infections are chronically tired. Fortunately, though, I have not yet seen someone who has both POTS and HIV. Might there be other long-term viral infections that show up as POTS?

During the past two decades, researchers have studied potential viral causes of chronic fatigue. There were hints that enteroviruses in the stomach, viruses originating in monkeys, and gammaretroviruses might each be responsible for chronic fatigue in humans. Careful research, though, has shown no such evidence, and we still know of no active infection that's responsible for chronic fatigue in adolescents.

It would be nice if a virus or other infectious agent could be found that was the cause of POTS and ongoing fatigue. So far, though, that is looking increasingly unlikely. Even though common infections may trigger the onset of POTS, there is no evidence that an active treatable infection accounts for people staying sick with POTS.

Immunity and autoimmunity

Evidence suggests a strong link between infection and the development of POTS. So it seems possible that infection triggers some sort of an immune response and that this triggered immune response is then responsible for POTS. Might this be true?

Science is pretty complicated. But as I've seen with my own children, young people these days are learning medical scientific information at a much earlier age than their parents, stuff that had hardly been discovered when I was in medical school.

When a human body is invaded by germs, its immune system responds by going into "attack mode." Part of the attack is to shoot "bullets"— antibodies to immobilize the germs. B-cells are the antibody-makers. Another part of the attack is to "take prisoners" by cleaning up and discarding the captured germs. T-cells are most responsible for this.

Along the way, "support staff" cells produce cytokines — chemicals that prime the body to respond to the invasion while hindering the advance of the invaders. Cytokines have names like tumor necrosis factor (TNF)-alpha, interferon-gamma and numerous interleukins followed by a number. Studies have shown that adolescents with chronic fatigue do have increases in anti-inflammatory cytokines and reductions in proinflammatory cytokines. This suggests that the bodies of chronically fatigued people are trying to downgrade the inflammation.

In addition to studying teens, scientists also have evaluated adults with chronic fatigue. Many tired adults have unusually low levels of natural killer T-cells, a special type of T-cell. Again, this suggests that tired people have "tired" or underactive infection-fighting systems. Unfortunately, stimulating increases in natural killer T-cells doesn't change the levels of fatigue in these people.

When the human body is stimulated to fight against invading germs, it sometimes produces lots of other antibodies in addition to those that are specific for the invaders. Occasionally, some of these antibodies actually attack the person's healthy parts instead of just attacking invading germs. When the body fights against itself, we call it autoimmunity. Autoimmune diseases include chronic conditions such as lupus and juvenile idiopathic arthritis.

In some early studies of adults with POTS, about 10% of participants had antibodies floating around their blood that were targeted against autonomic nerve receptors. This readily supported the theory that an infection might have caused an abnormal immune response that made the body attack its own nerve receptors, thus causing POTS. Unfortunately, this turns out to be, at most, a very small part of the story.

More than 90% of people with POTS do *not* have identifiable antibodies against their nerve receptors. And symptoms experienced by people with POTS — with and without the presence of these anti-receptor antibodies — look the same. It's not clear that the antibodies are actually causing trouble in most people with POTS.

There have been a few people with POTS who have elevated levels of autoantibodies. Giving anti-inflammatory treatments (such as intravenous immunoglobulin) to these patients has on some occasions been associated with improvement or even resolution of symptoms at the same time that antibody levels are dropping.

Wow! How do we put all of this together?

Clearly, people with chronic fatigue have some abnormalities in their immune systems. We don't yet know, though, if these abnormalities cause the fatigue or result from the fatigue — the old "chicken and egg" question of which came first. And, so far, there's no evidence that treating the immune irregularities alters outcomes for fatigued people. Among people diagnosed with POTS, there are a few with unusual antibodies and a rare few of those might respond to anti-immune treatment.

The biggest lesson from all of this immunity stuff is probably that we need to keep advancing the frontiers of science. Even though anti-immune treatment can't currently help many people with POTS, it could be that future research produces better treatments.

"Just" deconditioning

Remember Dr. Seuss' book about the Grinch who stole Christmas? Dr. Seuss' mythical Grinch had a heart "two sizes too small" and was so mean that he tried to stop Christmas from happening. In the end, he couldn't rob children of their Christmas fun, though, and his heart ended up growing as he joined in the community festivities.

What does the Grinch have to do with POTS?

A great POTS research team in Texas has suggested that POTS should be called the "Grinch syndrome" because, as they see it, the real problem is that people with POTS have shrunken hearts. No, people with POTS haven't lost their emotions or their Christmas spirit. It's just that some people with POTS seem to have physically smaller hearts.

Hearts get smaller when they're out of shape. Hearts grow bigger and stronger with conditioning. People with POTS sometimes are out of shape and have smaller hearts.

Remember the VO_2 max stuff we discussed in Chapter 5? In that chapter, we were talking mostly about muscle deconditioning. On a larger scale, though, the heart also can be deconditioned. Hearts can change in size with cardiac deconditioning.

About two-thirds of the adolescents with POTS that we see in Minnesota have cardiac deconditioning. But is their POTS due to deconditioning, or did their POTS make them so tired that they were less active and subsequently became deconditioned? Either explanation can be true. For some people, both explanations are true.

If POTS is solely due to deconditioning, then the total treatment will be to get reconditioned. And for some people, reconditioning is all it takes to get better from POTS.

But if POTS is only partly (or not at all) due to deconditioning, then something more than reconditioning exercise will be needed to recover. Our research is ongoing. Although most of our patients with POTS are deconditioned when we see them, this still doesn't tell us whether POTS or deconditioning came first. The other third of our patients with POTS are not deconditioned even though they have POTS.

The main characteristic of POTS seems to be that blood pools in the distant (peripheral) parts of the body and that the circulating blood volume decreases. This pooling of blood is due to abnormal changes in the nerve control of the tightness of the blood vessels. People with or without deconditioning can have biological evidence of altered blood flow and POTS.

So, can deconditioning all by itself look like POTS? Yes.

But can people with POTS be well-conditioned? Yes, we see many patients like that.

And can people have both POTS (with neurologically altered blood flow) and deconditioning? Yes, and this accounts for most of the people with POTS that we see.

Genetic, learned, or epigenetic? Yes, yes, and yes!

It would be easier if there was just one cause of POTS. But that doesn't seem to be the case. Truly, POTS is multifactorial, and the important factors balance in different ways in different people.

Some people have post-infectious POTS and are probably impacted more than other people by alterations in the immune system. Rarely, people with POTS have autoantibodies attacking their autonomic systems. Many people with POTS are deconditioned, but sometimes the deconditioning is more a result than a cause of POTS. And a rare few people with POTS have a single genetic defect or some predisposing genetic conditions.

Yes, the cause of POTS is complicated. But that shouldn't surprise us. Since even before I went to medical school, there have always been discussions about "nature versus nurture." Society wondered if people turned out the way they did because of their genes or because of their experiences. While it seemed that both nature and nurture were important, debates still continued as to which factor was most important.

Then, we entered the genetic revolution. We learned to identify and clone genes. We mapped entire genomes. We figured out how changes in genes led to changes in proteins, which led to changes in behavior. We debated whether moral preferences and criminal behaviors and athletic performance were matters of choice or of genetic programming. Genes seemed like they might be the answer.

At the same time, we realized that the majority of our genes didn't seem to be doing much. They didn't encode any specific proteins. Could 90% of our genetic material really be redundant waste?

No! Along came the field of epigenetics. The "extra" genetic material is really part of the control system that regulates which genes get expressed and how much they get expressed. And life experiences (including infections) exert epigenetic control over our genes.

Sure, there is some potential programmed into our genes, but the way that potential is fulfilled depends on how our epigenetic control is modified by life experiences and the environment.

What's even more fascinating is that we are now learning that some diseases depend not just on our genes and the epigenetic influences on our genes. Some diseases and even some parts of our immunity are altered by the pattern of germs living in our intestines. We all have trillions of bacteria living in our intestines. The pattern of bacteria, the "microbiome," varies with age, geography, dietary intake, and antibiotic use.

Already, we know that POTS is probably linked to both genetic and epigenetic situations. Maybe someday we'll even learn that POTS is partly initiated by diet and by the germs living in the intestines.

Science is fascinating and exciting. But we can't wait for new research to figure everything out. Now, it is time (finally!) to move on to a discussion of what we actually do to evaluate people with POTS. After that, we can get to the real fun — recovery!

Section 4: Evaluation and recovery

Chapter 10: Evaluation of teens with possible POTS

Let's get practical. Hopefully, your primary care doctor can recognize chronic fatigue as it's developing, can identify contributing factors and correct them, and can prevent you from needing to travel far away for medical care. But what if things weren't working? What would happen if you were chronically tired and came to see me?

My hope is that all of you reading this book won't have to come see me. I want you to be able to find resources and recovery without bothering to come to Rochester, Minnesota. But I'll tell you what might happen if you come to see me — then you can figure out ways to get what you need without having to take a long, time-consuming trip to the Upper Midwest of the United States. I'll tell you what might happen here just as an example, but I'm hoping things can work out quickly and effectively for you wherever you are.

Before your arrival

If you really thought you might need to come see me or one of my colleagues, our team would try to get to know you a bit before we set up appointments. We'd hear from you and your family, and we'd review your medical records. If we thought we had something to offer that others hadn't provided, we'd customize an itinerary for your time at Mayo Clinic.

And you might wait. Unfortunately, there are lots of tired teenagers in the world, and many of them come to Mayo Clinic for care. Regrettably, some people have had to wait more than a year for an appointment here. Our team is growing and we are working to reduce wait times. But even better than decreased wait times is the possibility of your getting better without needing to come here. Maybe this book will be a help to you!

An initial visit

Before we meet, you might be having lots of other thoughts and feelings. If you come in winter, you might be feeling very cold, and you'd quickly understand why our downtown section is designed to allow foot travel between a mall, hotels, and Mayo Clinic without ever going outside.

If you're from a mountainous area, you might be impressed with how flat southern Minnesota is. If you're from an urban area, you'd feel like you were arriving on a scene from *Little House on the Prairie* — small towns surrounded by farmlands with scenic lakes and rivers. (There is even a little house that has become a historical site near here, a place where Laura Ingalls Wilder lived on this prairie.)

When you get to Mayo Clinic, you might wonder if you're in the lobby of a high-class hotel. You'd see wide open areas and marble floors and staircases. You'd see tourists taking selfies in front of a world-famous glass-blown chandelier. You might hear the sounds of volunteers at the grand piano providing impromptu concerts. You might pause, gawk, and say "Wow!"

I see people coming to Mayo Clinic at the end of their proverbial ropes; they are desperate for help. When they come into the wide-open, well-decorated facilities, they start to relax. They realize they will be taken seriously. They appreciate the personal connections. They start sensing hope for recovery even before they get upstairs to see me. So soak in the atmosphere. Chat with the friendly volunteers in the lobbies. Savor the scenery. Feel the potential for recovery and healing.

Next, you'd arrive in the children's center lobby. Yes, even if you're a young adult, you'd get to enjoy the forest scenery in the child-friendly waiting room. A clinical assistant would invite you into a private room, perhaps a room with a great view of the town and surrounding countryside. You might even see a peregrine falcon on the ledge outside your window. The clinical assistant would check your height, weight, blood pressure and pulse, and then review your current medications.

Then, I or one of my colleagues would get to meet you. Welcome! We'd take time to hear your story in your words. We'd also have your parents chime in for additional outside perspective. We'd go through the whole story of your symptoms and your previous care, and we'd hear details of your past and family history. If you wanted, you'd have your parents around for most of the visit, but we'd want at least some time to hear from you by yourself.

Then, you'd get to change into a not-so-cool gown for your physical exam. We'd probably check your pulse in a couple of different positions over several minutes. Nothing should be painful or uncomfortable about all of this evaluation.

After sharing your story with us and letting us check you out, you'd get dressed again. Your parents would join us to talk through initial impressions and plans. We'd discuss just what other tests and subspecialty consults might help to get you fully poised for recovery. Then, you'd get a printed itinerary and head on your way.

Lots of tests and consults

Depending on how many unanswered questions there are about you, it might take a few days to get things sorted out. Here are some tests you might undergo.

Blood and urine tests We'd probably do some blood and urine tests to make sure other conditions — like iron deficiency, vitamin D deficiency, anemia, thyroid disease, kidney trouble, liver issues, inflammation, or hormone imbalance — aren't creating underlying issues.

If you have random episodes of your face turning red ("flushing"), we might do urine tests to rule out mast cell activation disorder. If we thought you might be one of the people with autoimmune antibodies affecting your POTS, we might draw blood to look for those antibodies.

If your symptoms started very early in life or if you have strange elevations in blood pressure, we might do tests of chemicals such as catecholamines and metanephrines to make sure there isn't some other imbalance masquerading as POTS. Some of the catecholamine tests would be done in a special endocrinology laboratory where they can sample your blood both while you're lying down and standing; other blood tests would likely be done in a location near our cool "forested" lobby.

If we were concerned that you weren't taking in enough salt, we might even do a 24-hour urine collection to see how much sodium you are putting out. (Yup, if you go to the mall that day, you'd need to take your "bucket" along so as not to miss collecting some of your urine.)

But blood and urine tests would probably not provide the final answer, and we'd want to do some other tests as well.

Autonomic function tests Most likely, we'd want to better characterize just how well (or poorly) your autonomic nervous system is actually working. You'd go down a few floors and through a hall to the autonomic laboratory. You'd probably spend about an hour there doing three parts of our autonomic testing.

First, we'd put some tingly tapes on you to see how your sweat nerves respond to stimulation. These superficial sweat nerves are representative of other autonomic nerves and give valuable information. About 15% of the teens with POTS that we see have abnormalities in sweat nerve responses. Less commonly, we'd do a thermoregulatory sweat test where we warm you up to about 100.4 degrees F while you're covered with a sweat-sensitive colored powder. This would show the pattern of sweat output in different nerve areas of your body.

Second, you would do some breathing exercises while we measure how your pulse and blood pressure adapt to variations in the pressure in your chest.

Finally, you would lie down to rest while we monitor your pulse and blood pressure. When you're stabilized and calm, the table would gently tilt up to a 70-degree angle. You'd relax for 10 minutes as we monitor you. We'd need to shorten the test if you almost faint with tilting. Fainting is uncommon but it can happen. All this autonomic information will be critically important as we pull together thoughts about whether or not you actually have POTS and just what your nervous system is doing.

Exercise tests Realizing that cardiac deconditioning interacts with POTS in many adolescents, we might also decide to do a cardiopulmonary exercise test. The way we do this is to have you take a bicycle ride — to nowhere. In the special exercise lab, you'd get hooked up to some circulatory and breathing monitors and then pedal against varying resistances on a stationary bicycle. This would help us identify any breathing restrictions or limitations and would help us see if your body subconsciously tries so hard to do well that you breathe at an abnormally rapid rate. We'd determine your VO$_2$ max to see how conditioned your heart and muscles actually are.

Other tests Beyond all of this blood, urine, autonomic, and exercise testing, there is a chance that we'd want to do an electrocardiogram to make sure you have no heart rhythm problem. We might also want to do a chest X-ray to rule out other heart and lung problems. And we'd do whatever other specific tests are indicated to sort through other peculiarities in your own personal story of fatigue.

Maybe that's all you'd need to do to allow us to sort things out for you. More likely, though, we'd call in reinforcements. You wouldn't need to see all of the 2,000 doctors I work with, but we might want you to see a few colleagues to help make sure we are identifying all relevant problems and coming up with all helpful treatments.

If you have unusual headaches, we might have you see a neurologist. If you have swollen sore areas of your muscles or joints (instead of "just" pain), you might see a rheumatologist. If you have toileting challenges or abdominal pains, you might see a gastroenterologist, urologist, or both. If pain is debilitating, we might involve an anesthesiologist who specializes in pain management and a physiatrist who specializes in physical medicine and rehabilitation. We'd probably have you see a psychologist, too — not because we think you have mental health problems but to give you some tools to help you with recovery from a frustrating condition. Depending on your other symptoms and concerns, we might get some other subspecialists involved.

Or maybe we won't need to do much of this at all. Maybe your situation is more straightforward. But whatever testing and consultation we do could take a couple of days. Some fatigued patients find the process tiring. Others find they actually start recovering while going through the process of having to get up and get active for all the medical care. Some even make new friends in the lobbies as they see other adolescents facing similar challenges.

An introduction to STEPS

If your initial results are suggestive of POTS, we'd probably schedule time for you to meet with one of our nurse educators. We might even invite you to join other patients and parents to get some group education about POTS and the recovery process.

You'd get some written information and possibly see a brief video. All of this would give you tangible ideas about what POTS is and how you can thrive while recovering from POTS.

We'd introduce you to a treatment program that we call STEPS. (Of course, you won't need that introduction since you will have already read this book by then!) We call the program STEPS because it's a reminder that when you have POTS, you need to advance one step at a time along the road to recovery. We realize that there are often mountain-like obstacles blocking your view of normal life. But we also believe that you can climb those mountains one step at a time.

What do the letters stand for in the STEPS program?

▶ "S" reminds you to increase your salt intake. Salt helps hold fluid in a floppy blood system to build blood volume and keep enough blood flowing even when some pools in the legs.

▶ "T" tells you to take in lots of fluids. We advise that patients with POTS drink so much fluid that their urine usually looks clear like water.

▶ "E" is the key to recovery from POTS — exercise! Exercise conditions your heart and blood vessels.

▶ "P" is for prescription medications that benefit many (actually most) patients with POTS along their way toward full recovery.

▶ "S" is the *et cetera* category. It's a reminder to go to school, get plenty of sleep, and take advantage of opportunities for social and psychological support.

Along the way, you'll realize that recovery is personal. You'll get an individualized plan to return to good health. But you might have to reset some priorities, as a good nurse reminds us.

➕ NOTES FROM A NURSE

Teens as well as parents want to be successful. I have heard success is in the eye of the beholder. What is success, do you believe in success, and do you believe you can achieve it?

Talking with many tired teens in our practice, we often hear stories of sacrificing sleep to get more studying completed in hopes of getting or continuing to get the best grades. But I often wonder, as a fellow overachiever, when is enough studying enough? And does studying actually produce success versus consistently getting nine hours of sleep, which can reduce fatigue and the feeling of "running on empty"? Getting enough sleep allows the brain to reboot like a computer, thus allowing the brain to be more efficient. It can be a difficult balance, and I have been challenged that I may not be aware of how important good grades are for teens in today's world. But I have witnessed the success of teens willing to commit to a routine and get the recommended amount of nightly sleep, in addition to balancing studies and still having fun with friends. It can be done, but it can be a very challenging part of recovery. I have also witnessed teens achieving straight A's and not being able to get out of the house or attend school, or work a job because of overwhelming fatigue. And I've heard stories of feeling "stuck" because while addressing one problem (getting good grades), there's also another problem (not being able to attend college or get a job because of overwhelming fatigue) blocking the journey. It is great to be able to achieve terrific grades by exercising the mind, but if the rest of the body is not exercised, and there is imbalance, then is this true success?

— Kay

A wrap-up visit

Finally, I or one of my pediatrician or nurse practitioner colleagues would see you after these days of testing and evaluation. Though you would have already heard some of the results and recommendations, this would be the time to pull everything together.

We'd go through the details of all of your test results. We'd congratulate you on all the stuff your body is still doing well, and we'd summarize the abnormal findings. This customized knowledge would then lead to your personalized recovery plan to get you moving down the road to recovery. You would not be obligated to cry or to hug. But after many years of suffering with fatigue, many of our patients are so relieved to be understood and to have a recovery plan that they do cry tears of joyful relief. And they do share hugs of gratitude.

So now you have had a "virtual" visit to see me and the place I work. Since you've done this virtually and since you are reading this book, you might be able to get a similar effective evaluation and care closer to home without the hassle of travel. So let's move on; let's discuss in detail the steps toward recovery.

Chapter 11: How to overcome POTS

Congratulations on getting this far in the book! If you skipped all the earlier chapters and started here, I commend you for your enthusiasm about moving forward with recovery. If, however, you got to this point by reading all the rest of the book, I commend you even more! You, reader, already understand as much about chronic fatigue and POTS as anyone else in the world. Your knowledge of how the body works (and doesn't work) with POTS provides you with ideas of what you need to do to recover. And your introduction to what would happen if you visited me professionally has already introduced the key points of a recovery program.

But none of this is enough. We now must translate our knowledge and our optimistic enthusiasm into tangible action. We need to build a solid foundation for your body so that your body is poised for recovery.

Whether an adolescent has chronic fatigue, autonomic dysfunction with orthostatic intolerance or POTS (or all of this together), the treatment plan is very similar. In fact, it's really just the medications that vary — the majority of the treatment interventions will be the same for all of these conditions.

Make a team

We must set up an appropriate context to facilitate recovery.

The"American dream"is often viewed as the opportunity to work hard and achieve great things, to "pull yourself up by your boot-straps" and move from "rags to riches." But people with POTS need to learn instead from the African proverb that"It takes a village."

A tired teenager understands the feeling of being down and out. No one, however, should be expected to heal himself or herself. It takes a team. We can't pull ourselves up alone. We need help.

Take, for example, a building that is being raised. We put scaffold-ing around the growing building to provide structure and support as it goes up. Or a young tree that's recently been planted. It's often supported with ties and stakes until it grows strong enough to stand on its own.

Similarly, people with POTS need a surrounding scaffold, a team of people who support and help frame their recovery. They should not be told to"just deal with it."

Yes, the person with POTS will have to work hard to recover. But the person with POTS also needs a team to help. Who will you invite to join your team, to work with you toward recovery? It's important to include only people who truly put your needs first. As we com-monly say at Mayo Clinic,"The needs of the patient come first."

Family Usually, parents and family are important. Everyone in the person's home should be educated about POTS and about recovery from POTS. Everyone at home can help with recovery.

Recent research studies have evaluated the dynamics between teens with POTS and their parents. The results indicate that the more parents encourage normal activities and matter-of-factly approach the disease, the more their teens get active and stay functional. On the other hand, the more parents "baby" their teens — encourage rest and provide special benefits for inactivity — the more the teens stay disabled. The more family members anticipate the worst possible outcomes (catastrophize), the more the person with POTS struggles. Inappropriate parental attitudes and behaviors don't cause POTS, but positive parental attitudes and behaviors can help facilitate recovery. You need "cheerleaders" encouraging positive action on your team, not "pillow-fluffers" keeping you comfortably compromised and inactive.

School staff We need to get school staff on the recovery team, too. I often ask former POTS patients to identify what they see as the key to their recovery. The typical answers are "Exercise, exercise, exercise" and "Go to school." Even when someone is tired and can't do everything, they should be encouraged to be active and to go to school daily. We recommend that you have a study hall at school. This is also a good time to skip advanced placement (AP) and honors classes while you work on improving your health. AP and honors classes create a lot more stress and homework, which tend to make health worse.

👥 LAURA'S PARENTS

We had two significant meetings and weekly interactions with the high school staff. We had a major meeting while searching for a diagnosis and another once we determined that Laura had POTS. Laura attended a large (2,000+ students), very diverse public high school. Laura was in charge of both of these meetings. We had Laura set an agenda beforehand and she led the meetings. Present for the meetings were her guidance counselor, who was our liaison with the school, her teachers, the school psychologist and the school nurse. We allowed Laura to determine what information she wished to share. Over the many months, from her initial symptoms to diagnosis, Laura shared literature on POTS, detailed her personal struggles in coping with POTS, and recommended concrete ways that the school staff could help her with her challenges. Her teachers mentioned how valuable the Mayo Clinic POTS information booklet was. They in turn were free to ask any questions. These were not "pity parties" but working meetings. They were open and honest discussions. As parents, we only chimed in when necessary. The result of these meetings was that Laura felt she could approach any one of these individuals during the school day and in turn they had a knowledge base of how to support her. There was no need to bypass Laura and come to us although they were welcome to contact us at any time as well. Laura had established herself as "in charge" and the school staff members were aware they could speak directly with Laura should the need arise. We intervened on just a few occasions. This was a very empowering approach for Laura and established her as the driver in the recovery process with many passengers along for the trip.

Primary care provider A doctor? Yes, anyone with POTS should have a caring, primary doctor (or nurse practitioner) to guide the medical aspects of recovery. The doctor should know about POTS, stay updated about POTS, and carefully consider treatment adjustments to help facilitate recovery. Specialists can help with details of medications and with management of various associated conditions that the person may have in addition to POTS. And many people with POTS find that a well-informed nurse practitioner or nurse educator can be extremely helpful; several of my former patients want to come back for further input — from the nurses more than from me! Usually, though, the key medical member of your team will be the primary care provider, who can coordinate medical input for you.

Mental health care provider Most people with POTS recover gradually. And recovery can be plagued with frustrating ups and downs. Just as sports teams use motivational psychologists to help them push toward championships, so people with POTS can usually benefit from regular contact with a psychologist or other therapist. And if the person also has anxiety or depression along the way, the mental health care provider can help with those problems, too.

Even if no psychological problems are present, most people with POTS can benefit from talk therapy strategies such as cognitive behavioral therapy (CBT). CBT can help a person with POTS cope with his or her symptoms and, eventually, overcome the symptoms. CBT has proven effectiveness in helping people with chronic fatigue.

In fact, the combination of exercise, regular academic activities, and CBT is much more important for recovery from POTS than is medication.

Other care partners In addition to family, school staff, doctors, nurses, and mental health care providers, many people with POTS also find great help from including a physical therapist, a life coach, or both on their recovery teams. The physical therapist can help with details of an exercise program, and the life coach can help with goal setting and problem-solving.

The biggest input of these people, though, is that they can serve as adult "accountability partners" to give some nonfamily motivation and encouragement to help the teen with POTS stick with a recovery program.

👥 LAURA'S PARENTS

There were many days when getting Laura to exercise became a nagging nightmare. She would be so exhausted and the last thing she wanted to hear from us was that she should go for a walk or head to the gym.

We found Shahadah, a personal trainer at our gym who was willing to work with Laura. Laura shared all the POTS literature and the Mayo physical therapy guidelines with the trainer. The trainer researched POTS and constructed a plan for working with Laura.

The best thing about having a trainer was that the sessions were goal oriented and the workouts added another event on the weekly calendar that not only met the exercise need but were social in nature as well. Together Laura and the trainer would set short- and long-term goals. A short-term goal may be the number of repetitions of a certain exercise in a session or the plan to move on to a set of heavier weights by the following week. Long-term goals might be to run a 5K in six months' time. Laura has always taken a goal-oriented approach to many aspects of her life and this trainer was a perfect fit.

Laura's personal trainer was exceptionally talented and very determined to impact Laura's life. She was demanding and had a great sense of humor. Shahadah significantly impacted Laura's mental health in addition to her physical health.

🏃 LAURA'S PARENTS

When people ask us why we think Laura was able to recover from POTS we point to one constant goal through all the years. Our focus could be summarized in our mantra, which is "Stay connected."

POTS can be very isolating. In order to keep the isolation to a minimum we chose to work hard at keeping key people in her life: people who cared about her and could support her recovery process.

For Laura this included people in all aspects of her life. At the time we saw this approach as staying connected, but in hindsight we recognize that this approach actually allowed our daughter some sense of control and structure.

Even though her POTS could run amok, her world had some constants and some significant relationships. These people helped Laura set goals, both long and short term. They helped her feel happy. They were strong individuals and had high expectations for Laura. They encouraged her and gave her hope.

[Mom now talking] I often comment about how Laura and I spent a lot of time together during her teenage years. In all honesty, more mother-daughter time than most teenage girls or mothers would ever think necessary. Having other people in her life gave Laura a much needed break from us. As parents we were so happy that Laura had other people in her corner.

It is a long road for the entire family of a POTS patient, and it is nice to have other truly supportive members on your recovery team.

👥 LAURA'S PARENTS

Initially, when Laura was feeling unwell and missing school, her friends were calling and stopping by the house to check in with her. However, as the search for a diagnosis dragged on and Laura spent more time at home, her connection with friends quickly declined. We tried to explain to Laura that there was no ill intent on her friends' part. They were simply carrying on with their lives as she would have had she not been ill. We worked very hard to keep Laura in school so that she could stay connected with her friends. Out of sight, out of mind is especially true with teenagers.

Organizing occasional movie nights with many of her friends at our house was a wonderful way for Laura to catch up with friends without expending a great deal of energy. Hearing the fits of laughter coming from our family room was music to our ears. Although, a word to the wise: When organizing such events it is really important to set time guidelines. Teenage girls do not leave unless you tell them it is time to go. Laura became very adept at saying come watch a movie at my house, but I need to be in bed by 10:00.

We think Laura learned a valuable lesson about friendship during her recovery period. Even though you have hundreds of friends on Facebook, most are superficial. One or two good friends is all you really need when the going gets tough. One friend, in particular, stood by Laura and supported her through POTS. She didn't give up on Laura.

➕ NOTES FROM A NURSE

Having autonomic dysfunction can be a very isolating experience for teenagers. Not only do teens with POTS find themselves feeling lousy with symptoms, by missing school (due to
illness or medical work-up) they oftentimes find themselves
being dropped from their social circles. Because of this, teens
are often driven online, searching to find others experiencing
similar symptoms. We often get asked for recommendations
for support groups. While there can absolutely be a benefit in
finding solidarity with a peer experiencing similar symptoms, I
caution my patients that support groups are only helpful if they
do things to encourage one another's recovery. Groups that
trade exercise tips, ways to increase water, or celebrate ac-
complishments can provide a much-needed boost during this
difficult time. However, caution needs to be used to ensure
that the dynamics of the group do not take a turn to the negative, as this will not encourage recovery. I tell my patients that
if the group turns into the "Debbie Downer Club" I want them
out of there. It is much better in that case to surround yourself
with friends who understand that you have medical issues,
but that the basis of your friendship does not rely on a shared
diagnosis.

— Jeannie

Support system *The Lone Ranger* was an old time television show even when I was a child. We don't have lone rangers conquering POTS or many other problems these days. Instead, it takes a team. So work from the very beginning of a POTS recovery program to set up a supportive team that can facilitate implementation of the recovery plan.

Friends And, of course, you need to keep your friends on your team. We also need to choose our sources of information. Friends are good as friends, but sometimes well-meaning friends can give us bad advice. Beware!

👤 LAURA

There is no way that I would have been able to recover from POTS without my incredible support system. I was surrounded by people who understood my situation, and helped me become the best version of myself that I could be. My parents were absolutely incredible. They encouraged me every step of the way, and didn't view me as a sick kid. On days that were particularly difficult, my mom and dad would offer to come to the gym with me so that I wasn't alone. They were always positive, and even when I was having a terrible day, our house was full of optimism. I also had a personal trainer who helped me get back on my feet. Exercise was extremely difficult for me at first, but I was always laughing through my workouts with her. We set goals for the week, and she would make me specific workouts for the days that we did not meet so that I was always sticking to the exercise plan. Thanks to her, I went from barely being able to walk to running a 5K in less than a year! I had a wonderful violin teacher who also knew about my diagnosis and supported me throughout my recovery. I loved my lessons with her because I could forget about how my body was feeling and simply get lost in the music. I also surrounded myself with a group of wonderful friends who supported me throughout this time. They didn't care that I had POTS, and kept me laughing and smiling throughout the school day. The most important thing for me was that my support system was extremely positive. They did not ask me how I was feeling every minute of the day, or pity me because I had POTS. To them, I was a normal teenager.

Maximize intake

The main problem associated with POTS is that blood flow is compromised by floppy blood vessels that don't tighten up enough in response to position changes. Since we can't perfectly correct the blood vessel muscle contraction, a key focus of our treatment is to generously fill the blood vessels so there will still be enough volume circulating even when the blood vessels are floppy and act like they aren't full enough. Remember the S and T of STEPS?

In other words, we can't zap POTS and instantly cure it. And we can't replace all of the intricacies of nerve control. What we can do, though, is compensate for POTS. We can fill our blood vessels so that there's enough blood volume to circulate even while an excessive amount of blood volume is pooling in the legs or abdomen.

Increasing blood volume won't cure POTS. But it will keep the blood flowing. And it can decrease fatigue, dizziness, and other POTS symptoms.

So, how should we increase blood volume?

Drink more fluid The best and safest way is to drink more fluid.

How much fluid should we drink? We should drink enough to fully maintain a maximal blood volume. We know we are there when our kidneys — assuming our kidneys work appropriately and don't have a separate problem — don't need to try to hold on to extra fluid. A couple of ways to do this would be to test how much urine we put out or measure the density of the urine.

More simply, though, we know we are drinking enough fluid when our urine looks clear and colorless, like water. If our urine looks yellow, that means that our kidneys are trying to hold back on fluid loss to support our blood volume. Our goal is to have clear-looking urine. Most people can have clear-looking urine by taking in a total of about 3 or 4 liters of fluid per day. A liter is about 30 ounces.

What about intravenous infusions of fluid? Quick bursts of intravenous fluids (especially salty ones like saline fluid) seem and feel dramatic. But the effect is the same as drinking a similar volume of a sports drink. Those who advocate intravenous fluids for POTS (and I don't) suggest a liter once or twice a week. That's the same as drinking a liter of a sports drink twice a week. So, there's not a big help from intravenous fluids for all the hassle it involves. And there is a medical risk. I've seen people get infections and life-threatening blood clots from intravenous lines used to give fluids for POTS. So I do not recommend them.

I can almost hear you saying, "But if I drink more, I'll just have to go to the bathroom more." That's right! And that's why it's not enough to only increase fluid intake.

Up the salt You also need to increase your salt intake. Your body will try to keep your salt levels in balance. So if you eat more salt, your body will hold on to more fluid, including in your blood vessels. By increasing salt intake, you'll hang on to the extra water you're drinking. In this way, you'll increase your blood volume.

How much salt? Simply put, people with POTS should eat as much salt as their taste buds can tolerate. Some people with POTS do this naturally, as if their bodies already know that they want more salt. One girl with POTS who lived on a farm admitted that she had been licking the salt block when she was caring for calves in the barn. Her body knew what it needed! Other POTS patients need to gradually increase their salt intake as their taste buds and stomachs learn to tolerate it.

If we wanted to be medically sure that the salt intake is adequate, we would measure sodium output. To do that, we collect all the urine the patient produces in 24 hours. If there are at least 170 milliequivalents (mEq) of salt produced in a day, then the person is taking in enough salt; if not, then salt intake should be increased even more.

What kind of salt should be used? It's sodium that matters, so any type of salt, including regular table salt, is fine. It's not necessary to use sea salt or combinations of various sorts of salt.

CAN COMPRESSION STOCKINGS HELP?

Another physical means of building blood volume is to wear compression stockings — up to the knees or even upper thighs. Compression stockings help squeeze the blood vessels to prevent swelling and to push blood back into circulation. Not uncommonly, people with POTS find these to be either too uncomfortable or too unsightly, but some people find them to be helpful in preventing pooling of the blood. If using compression stockings, choose ones that provide 15 to 30 mm Hg of pressure.

When should people with POTS eat their salt? All day long is fine. Many people find that the mornings are easiest if they start with a sugar-free salty sports drink first thing after waking up — even before getting out of bed. (Plan ahead, and leave the drink next to your bed the night before.)

Add salt to food, and choose salty foods. Within the limits of a healthy diet that maintains normal weight, people with POTS can enjoy salted crackers, pretzels, popcorn and nuts, and pickles.

Sports drinks can be used to increase salt intake while getting a nice flavor, but drinking lots of sugared drinks can damage teeth and cause excessive weight gain. So the focus should be on drinking lots of plain water daily. Caffeinated foods and drinks should be avoided since the caffeine stimulates the autonomic nerves in twitchy, poorly regulated ways.

What about salt pills? They're okay, but I prefer to be more "natural" and just have patients eat more salt. If someone chooses to use salt pills, three or four standard sports supplement pills containing about 250 milligrams (mg) can be used per day.

Only very, very rarely does a person with POTS take in too much salt. Puffy eyelids in the morning may be a sign of too much salt intake. If that happens, the person may need to cut back a little on salt intake.

Once POTS symptoms have been fully resolved for a few years, salt intake can be cut back. In the same way that increased salt intake helps people with POTS maximize their blood volumes, excessive salt intake in people without POTS can overfill the circulatory system and cause high blood pressure.

So for those who follow the STEPS in treating POTS (see page 145), we build blood volume by eating as much salt as our taste buds can tolerate and by taking in so much fluid that our urine looks clear like water. Many people find that these changes (along with exercise) are adequate to overcome the debilitation of POTS.

Move

Remember what I said earlier, about what patients have pointed out after they've recovered from POTS? They say a key to recovery is "Exercise, exercise, exercise." Do you want to recover from POTS? Then exercise!

Physical activity and exercise actually help our autonomic nervous system to relearn how to make blood flow properly. To "cure" POTS, exercise is the key. Fluid, salt, and medication help us do better along the way, but exercise helps us actually get better.

I can almost feel you sinking into depression as you read this. How can you exercise when you feel so tired? It's not like you want to just lie around doing nothing. You feel like your body can't exercise!

I hear you. I believe you. And I understand you.

But I also know that some of your nerves are confused and aren't regulating blood flow properly. Other nerves are confused and are telling you that you're too tired to exercise. We should not always believe what confused nerves are saying!

Astronauts returning from space have it relatively easy. They just need to gradually work back up to exercise for a couple of days. People with POTS have it harder; it takes months to get the nervous system working better. And POTS frequently puts people at risk of post-exertional fatigue. Exercise makes people with POTS feel more tired. So it's vitally important to plan an exercise routine that's consistent and gradually becomes more intense.

What kind of exercise is best? Someday, we'll have detailed answers about what exercise is best. But until more research is done, we advise what we think is best based on what we know.

Aerobic exercise is important. That's the "cardio" kind of exercise. We can get reconditioned by exercising in any position, but upright exercise is probably most effective in helping the body learn to circulate blood uphill against gravity.

If necessary, you can start with swimming or a recumbent bicycle and progress gradually to upright exercise, like walking briskly, biking on an upright stationary or outdoor bike, or using an elliptical machine. If you like jogging, you could eventually work up to that.

▲ LAURA

Exercise was the key to my recovery. It felt like an insurmountable goal. I was so incredibly tired. How was I supposed to exercise? Having a personal trainer was extremely helpful for me. At first, I didn't know how vigorously to exercise, so it was beneficial to have someone making workouts for me to do every day. There will be days that you don't think you could possibly exercise. Do it anyway. On particularly bad days, when I didn't know how I would get through a full day at school, exercise, and finish my homework, I used to imagine how proud I would be of myself when I was going to bed at the end of the day, knowing that I had accomplished my goals. I would hold onto that feeling throughout the day, pushing myself to get through minute by minute.

Here's the thing about POTS recovery: It doesn't happen overnight. You don't exercise for a day and magically feel better. So in my mind, if I was going to feel sick either way, I might as well do the things that I knew were helping me move forward. So go to school. Even if you feel absolutely terrible. You might think to yourself, "No one understands. If they knew how sick I felt, they would realize why I can't make it to school today." I understand. There are kids with POTS all over the world who understand. That doesn't mean you get to take the day off. Because in the long run, watching Netflix on your couch and feeling sorry for yourself isn't going to aid in your recovery. In my experience, it's better to feel sick at school with your friends than alone on your couch. Push yourself to do things even when your body feels like it is working against you. Because one day, it doesn't feel so difficult. Waking up and getting to school no longer feels like such a challenge. It gets better.

You will rarely see me without a water bottle nearby. I hydrate like it is my job. In high school, I told my teachers that hydration was a key point in my recovery, and asked that I be allowed to excuse myself to the restroom whenever needed. My go-to snack during the school day was extremely salty popcorn — the more salt, the better! I drank a Gatorade before getting out of bed in the morning, and would do squats and bicep curls before getting ready for school. This helped me wake up and feel prepared to conquer my day.

How hard should your aerobic exercise be? We shouldn't be pushing so hard that we overdo it, but we should be working intensely enough to be working. Some people like to adjust the intensity of exercise based on reaching a target heart rate (usually 220 minus your age in years times about 0.7; that comes to about 145 for the average teenager).

The trouble is that the heart rate isn't completely reliable in people with POTS — some reach their target heart rate just by standing up, holding still! So I usually advise my patients to exercise at an intensity that makes them breathe a bit faster than normal but not too fast. They should still be able to carry on some semblance of a conversation and also get sweaty. The speed of the activity will increase with conditioning, but the goal is still to be breathing a bit faster than normal.

How often should you exercise? Most importantly, exercise should be regular. I suggest exercising six or seven days each week. Most people with POTS are more tired in the morning, and most people find it hard to fall asleep if they exercise right before bedtime. So late afternoon usually works well for a daily session of aerobic exercise for someone with POTS.

For how long should you exercise? The eventual goal is to get up to 30 minutes of sustained exercise each day (six or seven times each week). But be reasonable! Start small and then build up slowly. I've had some patients who are so debilitated that it takes a week or two to be able to get out of bed. Usually, though, people can tolerate at least five minutes to start. The duration of exercise can then be increased by a minute or two every four days. At that rate, you would successfully reach your 30 minute goal after just a month or two.

If you're drained and tired the day following your initial exercise sessions, you probably pushed it for too long. You should start with a duration of exercise that doesn't leave you more tired than usual the next morning. If you start with too much exercise and get stuck in bed the next day or you can't go to school, you know that you started with too much exercise!

What if you're sick? POTS symptoms increase when you're sick with colds or other illnesses. So the most important time for exercise is when the body is getting worn down by an illness. If, however, you have a fever, you can back off on the exercise. Otherwise, it's best to exercise through illnesses without a fever.

EXERCISE IS THE KEY TO RECOVERY FROM POTS. Repeat this regularly, like a mantra. Live this out daily. Exercise! Aerobic, upright exercise every day (well, at least six days each week) is the key to recovery from POTS.

But that's not all! In addition to the daily exercise session, there are other ways you can move and care for your body to help reduce the symptoms of POTS.

Additional physical activity Strive to add at least another half hour each day of additional physical activity. This can be the routine or fun stuff — participating in physical education at school, walking the dog, shooting hoops, doing yoga or martial arts, or strength training. The eventual total daily activity should be for at least an hour a day, but you'll be working up gradually to your half hour of daily aerobic exercise along with 30 minutes of other activity. Strength training is an important activity to do about three times a week on nonconsecutive days. Ask your physical therapist to give you a plan. You could also hire a personal trainer at your local gym for one to two sessions to give you a strength training plan.

Morning muscle work One other kind of exercise can help you feel better, too. In the morning, your POTS-compromised body will feel most tired as you get up and try to get going. Many teenagers with POTS find that it helps to do some big muscle exercises first thing after getting up. This doesn't cure anything, but the muscle squeezing causes the blood vessels to push the blood into circulation.

For about two minutes, you can do a few repetitions of big muscle exercises each morning. The goal is to get the blood flowing, not to tone or strengthen the muscles. You can start with bicep curls — holding 2 to 5 pounds in your hand and then flexing the arm at the elbow to pull your hand up toward your shoulder. You can do that 20 times with each arm. Then you can do squats — squatting into a crouched position and then standing up, again about 20 times. If the squatting and rising makes you dizzy, you can do toe stands (going up and down from tip-toes) or kicking (while sitting, with something that weighs a few pounds in a sock draped over your ankle) instead.

Plenty of sleep At the same time, exercise needs to be balanced with adequate sleep. People with POTS rarely sleep well. We can help by selecting a calming evening environment. Caffeine should be avoided. Technology and devices should be turned off an hour before bedtime. The awakening time should be programmed, and then the bedtime can be adjusted to allow adequate sleep prior to awakening to allow teens to get 8.5 to 9.5 hours of sleep each night. Naps should be avoided. Structuring sleep habits leads to improved sleep quality and quantity.

Motivation and direction

There are lots of aspects of treatment for people with POTS. We started by saying "It takes a team," and we finish this treatment section with the reminder that we need to help ourselves stay motivated. Recovery requires difficult, uncomfortable work every day. We need to be encouraging throughout the process.

A favorite quote among my POTS patients is, "When you can't see the light at the end of the tunnel, get up and walk down there and turn the light on yourself." POTS can be overwhelmingly discouraging at times. We don't always feel like getting up and getting going. Yet we must keep moving forward. Stop the pity party. Go for recovery!

How can we help ourselves stay motivated? Daily encouragement helps — but encouragement should be real. We should identify specific successes (like following the treatment plan, even if the

GO TO SCHOOL

One of the best ways to facilitate physical recovery with POTS is to go to school. This is very difficult for severely affected individuals, but it's vitally important. The physical activity and structure of school do a lot to help the body regain physical ability as the autonomic nervous system is stimulated to recover. Even if you feel too tired to think much at school, it's important to physically participate in school activities to help the body recover. Academic "catch up" can take place at home later in the day. For the body's sake, I agree with former POTS patients who tell me to urge current patients to "Go to school. Whether you feel like it or not, go to school!"

physical feelings aren't great). We shouldn't nag for progress but congratulate for good steps being taken. We should keep the end in sight, realizing that almost all teens with POTS do eventually fully recover. We should set reasonable goals and tolerate our physical limitations. We should prioritize activities and the use of limited energy so that the most important things are accomplished.

A healing mindset

Research and experience in North America and Europe demonstrate that cognitive behavioral therapy (CBT) is extremely effective both in facilitating function with chronic fatigue and in promoting recovery from chronic fatigue and POTS. A skilled CBT-trained psychologist

As a family we worked hard to keep life as positive as possible. Whenever Laura would have a challenging doctor's appointment or test we would frequently follow the appointment with lunch at City Market where she would enjoy a heaping bowl of mac 'n cheese. On the way to these appointments Laura would often comment that she was feeling okay because she knew there would be mac 'n cheese when it was all over. Recently I was at City Market with some friends and I texted her a picture with a heart emoji. It was proof that even some of her most difficult days had some positive and hopeful moments.

We tried hard to keep life as normal as possible. We still went on vacation. We still went to the movies. Life carried on as best we could. Don't lose sight of your goals. "Get off Facebook" and "live your own life" were two phrases that were repeated several times in our house when Laura would be having a bad day.

Laura never joined in on any of the various websites for people with POTS. Laura knew what she had and what she needed to do to move forward. She needed to focus on her own recovery and not get caught up in comparing herself with others with the same condition. This was one way of staying away from a pity party.

___

can teach techniques to help put the mind back in control of even the "involuntary" nervous system.

Biofeedback training helps a person learn how to control even involuntary bodily functions like temperature regulation and heart rate. Deep diaphragmatic breathing can help reprogram relevant nerves to resolve nausea and vomiting. Thought training can help develop habits of positive, recovery-promoting, health-stimulating thoughts. I even retrained my body to help me actually enjoy going uphill against the wind when I jog. I convinced myself that it is easier on my knees to go uphill than downhill, and it is easier to stay cool when the wind is blowing at me — both are true, and focusing on those truths helped me keep running. Otherwise, I was focusing on "poor me, it's so hot, and it's hard to run uphill" thoughts that made it hard to keep moving forward. I've had POTS patients with such severe eating troubles that they had feeding tubes placed surgically; cognitive behavioral therapy got them eating tube-free, within just a couple of weeks.

And we should stay in touch with others. Millions of teenagers have POTS and almost all end up doing well. Research has proven good outcomes in the vast majority of people with adolescent-onset POTS. We should stay in touch with others who can encourage us onward, and we should avoid those who drag us down. We should focus on functioning and give minimal attention to our physical feelings.

POTS is bad enough. Adding inactivity and noncompliance to treatment on top of POTS is tragic. We must keep stepping forward as we move onward on the road to recovery.

Get the idea? You can recover from autonomic dysfunction, orthostatic intolerance, and POTS by changing your fluid and salt intake, exercising regularly, minding your schedule, and getting cognitive behavioral therapy. But, sometimes, especially for adolescents with POTS, medications can help, too, as long as you're doing everything else to facilitate recovery. So keep reading; lots of details about medication for patients with POTS are waiting for you in the next chapter.

Chapter 12: Possible medications

Medications don't cure POTS. The cure for POTS comes with time and exercise. Along the way, people with POTS function better when they build up their blood volume, get good sleep, follow balanced daily schedules, and fortify their minds with cognitive behavioral therapy. What good are medications?

Remember, exercise is the key, and increased fluid and salt intake is essential. Medication use is less important than the fluids, salt, and exercise.

But most people with POTS can benefit from medication in addition to these other measures. Medication is a bit like the steering wheel of a car — it can help you head in the correct direction, but it won't cause progress unless you are already moving (by exercising) and have a full tank (by taking in lots of fluids and salt).

The main usefulness of medications for POTS is to tighten up muscle tone around blood vessels and intestines so as to increase flow. The three main chemical means of increasing flow involve targeting neurotransmitters toward beta receptors, alpha receptors, and serotonin receptors. After reviewing these, I'll mention some other medications that have also been used.

Beta blockers

To function appropriately, blood vessel muscles depend on nerve impulses that tell them when to constrict and when to relax. "Constrict" messages activate alpha receptors on blood vessel muscle cells, while "relax" messages activate beta receptors. Many adults use beta blockers for heart disease and high blood pressure. These medications decrease the heart rate but also keeps blood vessels from relaxing too much. Beta blockers can help people with POTS in a similar way — by preventing blood vessel muscles from over-relaxing and improving blood flow. Practically speaking, beta blockers are the medication that patients feel helps them most with POTS symptoms.

There are several different beta blockers, and they vary in terms of effect and side effects. Metoprolol is my personal first choice as a beta blocker for POTS. I prescribe the regular form since the long-acting form doesn't seem to work as well for POTS symptoms. I usually give teenagers 25 milligrams (mg) twice during a day; the first dose can be taken 15 to 20 minutes before getting out of bed in the morning, and the second dose is taken with lunch. Occasionally, some patients need a late afternoon dose or larger doses. For adults, propranolol is effective for POTS, even in low doses. Some teenagers, though, get overly fatigued on propranolol. Atenolol and nadolol are other good options as oral beta blockers.

Each beta blocker dose works for about four to eight hours, so there's no need to build up or wean down on doses. But the helpful effects aren't always obvious over the short-term, so beta blockers should be tried for at least a month before giving up on them.

Theoretically, beta blockers can make asthma worse, but this is rarely an issue in practice. Nonetheless, if someone with asthma and POTS uses a beta blocker, it's important to monitor for worsening asthma symptoms, which might require a change in beta blocker use.

Mast cell activation disorders are rare. But they can either look like or complicate POTS. And people with mast cell activation disorders might get worse on beta blockers. So if someone seems to have POTS but gets clearly worse on beta blocker treatment, especially if he or she experiences random facial flushing, I'd think about doing a urine test that checks for the substances N-methylhistamine, leukotriene and prostaglandin to rule out a mast cell activation disorder.

👤 LAURA

I was prescribed a beta blocker when I was diagnosed, and it helped me throughout my recovery. With the beta blocker, my heart wouldn't race as much, and I felt more comfortable throughout the day.

Midodrine

In addition to blocking the "relax" messages, we can also augment the "constrict" messages with midodrine. This medication is usually used three times each day, starting at 2.5 mg per dose and increasing every week or two by 2.5 mg per dose up to 5 mg (or even 10 mg, if needed) by mouth three times daily.

The temperature-regulating skin nerves of some people get over-stimulated on midodrine; that's why we start patients on a low dose and build up gradually. Usually, the creepy-crawly, goose bump-like feelings fade after a day or two, and the dose can be continued. If the skin feelings are too bothersome, though, the dose can be reduced. (One patient told me that he liked the effect. He thought it felt like a continuous scalp massage.)

The other potential side effect with midodrine is that it increases blood flow too much when the person is lying down. This can cause headaches. So midodrine should not be taken within about four hours of lying down (which is to say, avoid evening doses). And midodrine can cause high blood pressure when lying down.

Of course, medication doses should be customized for each individual by a doctor who's responsible for the patient's care. I offer my general dosing guidelines only as a reference, not to dictate any particular doctor's prescribing habits. Some doctors prefer to give midodrine much more frequently — four to six times per day. I haven't found this to be effective.

Serotonin

Many people have heard of the brain chemical serotonin since it's often linked to depression. A big function of serotonin is to transmit signals between nerve cells. Medications that boost serotonin levels and improve nerve communication are called selective serotonin reuptake inhibitors (SSRIs). SSRIs are commonly prescribed for depression. What is lesser known is that serotonin also is produced along the intestinal tract, even more so than in the brain. Taking an SSRI can help smooth out intestinal flow and, to some degree, blood flow in people with POTS. I often add an SSRI to the treatment regimen if a patient with POTS has lots of gastrointestinal symptoms and isn't improving enough on metoprolol and midodrine.

Any of the SSRIs available should be fine, but there has been helpful research on citalopram for adolescents with chronic abdominal pain. So I usually select citalopram as my first choice of an SSRI medication. Doses are typically the same as for treating depression. SSRIs are usually taken at bedtime since they sometimes make people sleepy; some people, though, feel less sleepy after an SSRI dose and choose to take it in the morning.

A related form of medication is the serotonin and norepinephrine reuptake inhibitor (SNRI). Like serotonin, norepinephrine is a chemical messenger that helps nerve cells communicate. But using an SNRI instead of an SSRI doesn't seem to make much difference for people with POTS. While not much research has been done on medications in adolescents with POTS, we do know that the SNRI duloxetine has been useful for pain in adults with fibromyalgia.

Of course, SSRIs and all other medications should be used cautiously. Rarely, depressed individuals have felt empowered enough (but still not less depressed) to act on their depression and take their own lives. It's not clear that this would be a risk for someone using an SSRI for POTS.

Other POTS medications

Other medications that might help ease POTS symptoms include:

Fludrocortisone This drug is a steroid-related medication that tricks the kidneys into holding on to more fluid and salt; these are desirable effects for people with POTS. Side effects are uncommon, but dangerous salt imbalances have been reported. My personal preference is to have patients drink lots of fluids and eat lots of salt and not bother with fludrocortisone. Many doctors who treat POTS, though, like to use fludrocortisone.

Ivabradine This is a medication that's been used in Europe for several years, mostly in adults with heart failure but also in some people with low blood pressure. It is increasingly used for POTS in Europe and has been used some for adolescents with POTS in the U.S., especially those with very rapid heart rates. Ivabradine might turn out to be very effective, but data are still lacking on both safety and effectiveness in children and adolescents.

Stimulants Rarely, attention deficit stimulants like methylphenidate and amphetamines have been reported to help people with POTS think more alertly, but they haven't been well-studied as a treatment for POTS.

Modafinil is a mild stimulant used by long-haul truck drivers and shift workers to help them keep awake at night. It's expensive but it occasionally has been reported to help some people with POTS feel less fatigued. I hardly ever prescribe these stimulants for patients with POTS, but some doctors do.

Pyridostigmine This is a medication that's useful for different nervous system conditions. Studies indicate it can be helpful in some adults with POTS. I have only used it in a few adolescents with POTS, but it seems to help some that have particularly severe intestinal or bladder problems due to POTS.

Erythropoietin This is a kidney chemical that stimulates increases in blood volume and in the production of red blood cells. Some people have advocated prescribing erythropoietin for POTS, but I have no experience with it and don't recommend it.

Antiperspirant Excessive sweating is a physical and social challenge for some people with POTS. A prescription-strength antiperspirant can be tried. A couple of my patients have found the drug oral glycopyrrolate to be helpful. But there's not enough experience with it in the context of POTS to know if it's worthwhile.

Medications for associated conditions

Many people with POTS have associated conditions, such as low iron or chronic pain. Sometimes, medications can help address these other problems.

Iron deficiency About half of our patients with POTS have low ferritin levels, which is indicative of iron deficiency. Iron supplements are recommended, about 4 to 5 mg of elemental iron per kilogram of body weight divided into two or three doses per day; this translates to about 65 mg of elemental iron (about the amount found in a 325 mg ferrous sulfate pill) by mouth three times daily.

If the person has restless legs syndrome, the goal is to get the ferritin level up over 50 nanograms per milliliter (ng/mL); if the person doesn't have restless legs syndrome, I aim at getting the ferritin level up to at least 20 ng/mL.

Iron is better absorbed if taken with vitamin C. In addition, iron can be constipating, so increased fluid and fiber intake and laxatives might be necessary.

Vitamin D deficiency Nearly a third of our patients with POTS have low vitamin D levels, which has been associated with chronic pain. If the vitamin D level is less than 20 ng/mL, I suggest once-daily oral supplements — about 1,000 International Units (IU) per dose, with more for heavier people and for people with very low levels.

If either the ferritin or vitamin D level is low, I repeat the blood test after a couple of months of treatment to make sure we have corrected the problem. I then keep treatment going for many months to prevent the level from dropping again.

Chronic pain Many people with POTS have chronic pain. Sometimes, SSRIs and SSNRIs can help with chronic pain.

Narcotics help only briefly and make it harder to actually overcome the pain; they shouldn't be given to people with POTS for chronic pain. Narcotics are fine for a couple of days after an injury or operation, though.

Amitriptyline and nortriptyline, which belong to an older group of antidepressants, can be useful for chronic pain in some people with POTS, as can gabapentin, which is also used for seizures.

Insomnia Sleep is a real problem for many patients with POTS. I only prescribe sedatives (like zolpidem) for very brief time periods for travelers experiencing jet lag. I do not recommend sedatives for patients with chronic tiredness.

Sometimes, melatonin (3 to 5 mg in the evening) helps initiate sleep, and it seems safe. Amitriptyline can also help with sleep in some people with POTS, but it can alter the sweat responses on autonomic nerve testing.

Anxiety or depression As we've mentioned, the neurotransmitters that relate to POTS also relate to anxiety and depression. (Beta blockers are even used for performance anxiety, also known as stage fright.) If a person with POTS needs medications for anxiety or depression, he or she might find that SSRIs do double duty in also helping with the POTS itself.

On the path to recovery

Wow! That's a lot of medications. Some people with POTS do fine with just nondrug treatments, but many do need at least a beta blocker (or midodrine). Some end up on both a beta blocker and midodrine, and a few need those as well as an SSRI, such as citalo-pram. In my experience, it's uncommon for people with POTS to need more than a couple of medications, but care should always be customized to best serve the individual patient.

Now, then, people with POTS have tools for recovery. They build up blood volume with increased fluid and salt intake. They do aerobic exercise every day. They get adequate sleep and keep regular schedules so their bodies are primed for good functional restoration. They use their minds, with the help of cognitive behavioral therapy, to better control and regulate bodily functions. They use medications, as appropriate, along the way. And they recover!

All this recovery stuff is great, but it takes time. During the long road of hard work toward recovery, well-meaning friends (and internet sources) might offer a distraction from forward progress. So remember to think clearly, even during the long, hard days and nights of recovery.

Chapter 13: Placebos and distractions

I hope you've followed everything we've been sharing together in this book. I know some of this is complicated, and I've used some big words. At the same time, I'm just a pediatrician. I tend to think simply. I talk about "ear thingies" instead of otoscopes and "circle things" instead of stethoscopes. My patients tend to use bigger words than I do. So I hope all this nervous system stuff has been intelligible.

I know that my POTS patients, and their parents, are usually very bright and read a lot. So I'd like to use a medical article as an example of how I'd advise that we all keep learning from science. There are at least four lessons we can learn from a classic research article.

Clare McDermott is a researcher in Southampton, England, who works with a team to better understand and treat people with chronic fatigue syndrome. She and her team realize that a gradual increase in exercise along with cognitive behavioral therapy is the only proven means of overcoming chronic fatigue, but they also seek to find new treatments that might be helpful.

Remember how we said that people with chronic fatigue seem to have suppressed levels of natural killer T-cells? The McDermott group tried to decrease fatigue by increasing the levels of these natural killer cells. This made sense, and there had been an earlier report suggesting that fatigued patients might feel better if they took arabinoxylane, a natural killer T-cell stimulant.

So in order to test the value of this medication, Dr. McDermott and her colleagues conducted a randomized, controlled, double-blind study — in other words, a well-designed trial — of 71 patients. Let's see what happened.

Lesson #1
Look before you leap

Chronic illness attracts compassion. People want to help. And tired teenagers (and their parents) seem to receive lots of well-intentioned advice. Other people, even strangers, have heard about supposedly similar problems and want to share news about things that might help. Tired teenagers can expect to hear lots of well-motivated input about what they should do to get better.

Between friends, relatives, and the internet, how should you respond to new suggestions about what you should do? Like the British researchers, you should check things out carefully. Some people had reportedly been helped by using arabinoxylane to stimulate natural killer T-cell production, and it was reasonable to think that this treatment would also help others. But instead of simply starting to prescribe arabinoxylane, these researchers decided to investigate it further. They checked it out. Like the old adage says, you should "look before you leap" — check things out before committing.

Especially with medical interventions, it's important to not jump too quickly. No medication is perfectly safe, and you need to be sure that the benefits outweigh the risks.

If you do a Google search on the term *chronic fatigue treatment,* you'll likely find about two million relevant sites. How do you choose where to look and what to check out?

It helps to have a trusted medical professional, such as your doctor, involved who can direct you to up-to-date therapies. It also helps to connect with people who have had similar troubles. If you hear of a treatment that's reported to help and that seems to make sense, then maybe you can check it out — either by reading reliable resources or by talking to a doctor who is willing to help you understand it.

So Dr. McDermott and her group decided to check out arabinoxylane. They identified 34 patients who met the definition of chronic fatigue syndrome as provided in the 1990s by the Centers for Disease Control and Prevention. The patients were given a daily dose of arabinoxylane and repeatedly filled out questionnaires about how they were feeling. The researchers did careful statistical analysis of the results.

Lesson #2
Make sure it's relevant

Are you getting excited to hear about the results of the McDermott study? Perhaps you feel run down, and you feel like you get infections more often than your friends do. You believe what we've said about natural killer T-cells, and you wonder if this medication would work for you.

But I interrupted the story. Before telling you the results, I inserted another lesson. That's the way it is in real life. Before jumping ahead to the conclusions, we need to make sure that the research in question will apply to us. This was a study conducted in Britain, and people might be different there than they are where you live. It was also a study of adults who had a mean age of 42 years. Clothes and music preferences and schedules and just about everything else is different between people in their 40s and teenagers. Clearly, what works in 42-year-olds might not work the same way in teenagers.

Even if the medicine helps people the age of your parents, it might not help you. And maybe you have POTS. Lots of people with chronic fatigue have POTS, but these researchers didn't differentiate between people with POTS and people with chronic fatigue.

So back to our story.

In people who took arabinoxylane daily for eight weeks, physical fatigue scores decreased from 15.5 to 14. In addition, physical well-being scores improved from 37.7 to 40.8. These results don't look miraculous, but they do show an improvement of 10% over just two months.

Lots of my patients would be thrilled to feel 10% better just by swallowing medicine daily for two months. And we know that teens are resilient and are more likely to recover from chronic fatigue than adults are. Maybe the medicine would work better in teenagers. We might even extrapolate the data to think that the 10% gain over two months would continue additively to provide a full cure over 20 months.

Ready to try this new product? Ready to go buy some medicine and boost your energy by 10%?

Lesson #3
The placebo effect

A placebo, also known as a "sugar pill," is something inactive that is used in research studies. It serves as a comparison to the treatment researchers are studying. Wise researchers like those in the McDermott group know that medication trials should include placebos as a benchmark. Otherwise, it's hard to know if the 10% improvement in symptoms was actually due to the medication or to some other factor.

In addition, we know that about a third of people taking placebos will think they get better, regardless of the study underway. This is called the placebo effect.

So the McDermott researchers got two bits of placebo-related information.

First, people filled out surveys about how they felt when they signed up for the study and then again when they were ready to start taking the medication (and again as the study progressed). Right away, the researchers found that fatigue scores had improved by about 10% just by signing up for the study. The participants had yet to take any medication, whether the placebo or the experimental drug.

Second, the study participants were divided into two groups. One group of 34 people got the experimental drug, arabinoxylane. The other group, consisting of 30 individuals, got the placebo. Subjects were randomly assigned to get either medication or placebo, and neither the subjects nor the researchers knew who was getting what (until they broke the code at the end of the study). In people who got the placebo, fatigue dropped by about 14% and overall sense of physical well-being improved by 14%. Even though the improvement was not significantly different between treatment and placebo groups, the placebo almost looks better than the treatment. This means that real arabinoxylane is no better than sugar pills of fake arabinoxylane.

So just because someone feels better after a treatment does not mean that the improvement is due to the treatment. Lots of other things are going on at the same time that might affect the symptoms, and the simple belief that the treatment will help can end up actually helping.

Lesson #4
Support matters

Why did people already start getting better before they took the medication? They were being seen regularly by experts, and the experts were listening as the participants described their symptoms and feelings. They were also exposed to optimism that perhaps the medication would help.

The final lesson is this (and this may apply more to parents and doctors): Let's harness those attributes of treatment programs; let's build a placebo effect into our care even if we don't take a placebo medication. Regardless of whatever we're providing for treatment, chronically tired teens should be listened to. They should have regular contact with their recovery team members, including doctors. Seemingly simple listening can actually help. They should be reminded with true optimism that data show that most chronically tired teenagers, even those with POTS, do recover.

Yes, most teenagers with POTS do recover. Will "most" include you? We discuss that in the next chapter.

Chapter 14: Optimism about the future

Chronic fatigue is, by definition, chronic. It lasts a long time. What should you expect if you have (or your child has) chronic fatigue? What is the outlook for people with POTS?

No one can accurately and definitively predict the future for any individual person, but there are several types of evidence that allow us to predict favorable outcomes with confidence. Some of the evidence comes from experience, and some comes from actual scientific data.

In this chapter, we review what we know about the prognosis for chronically tired teenagers. And — spoiler alert — we see that almost every teenager with chronic tiredness can function better, and the vast majority of tired teenagers, even those with POTS, recover and move forward in successful lives.

No crystal ball

But why is it so hard to predict outcomes for tired teenagers?

Part of the challenge is that every person is unique. Some teenagers are tired because they need more sleep or they need more iron.

They can get better quickly if they deal with the problem causing their tiredness. Some tired teenagers mostly need help to manage a mood disorder (such as depression or anxiety) and will then function lots better. Others have chronic fatigue with otherwise normal test results, and some even have POTS. For these teens, we know what to do for treatment, but outcomes take time.

Also, we science-minded people haven't accurately followed details of enough patients for enough years to really know how everyone does. There are only a handful of POTS research studies that compare medical treatments while following patients for more than a week. We know how hundreds or even thousands of patients have done, but some have neither stayed in touch to report progress nor been identified for follow-up studies. And even if we did know how all the last ten thousand patients did, we don't know which of those patients is most predictive of the outcome of any particular current patient.

So it's hard to accurately predict the future.

Evidence of recovery

But we do have a pretty good general idea of how people will do.

In my experience as a doctor, I've seen lots of tired teenagers recover completely and go on to thrive in life — even those without specific, easily treated lab abnormalities. Full recovery is absolutely possible.

But I've also seen a few teenagers who continued to require medical treatment for POTS longer than others and who struggled through their college years and into graduate school. Most of these teenagers improve, some fully recover, and some keep struggling for a while. But what does that mean for you? What sorts of percentages can be used to predict outcomes?

In 2009, we reported a survey of patients we had seen with fatigue and dizziness. Of those with POTS treated with a beta blocker, 100% said their symptoms had improved since their initial visit. This is very encouraging, even though we don't know about outcomes in those patients who didn't respond to the survey.

In 2012, some of my Mayo Clinic colleagues reported on 58 young adults (including a few adolescents) they had followed for a year. Twelve months after their initial diagnosis of POTS, symptoms were improved, and 37% no longer had enough postural tachycardia to qualify for a diagnosis of POTS. This first published report of outcomes of POTS was encouraging in that patients were improving after just a year, and more than a third of them no longer actually had POTS.

A few years later, we got fresh survey results back from 172 of our adolescent POTS patients an average of five years after we had initially seen them for POTS. Nearly three-fourths of them said that their health was at least "good" by then; 86% of them reported that their symptoms were either resolved or improved or only occurring intermittently. Most of those over age 18 years at the time of the study had started college, and about half of those over 23 years of age at the time of the survey had completed college. Yes, we have decades of evidence that teenagers and young adults with POTS can recover.

Some of our POTS patients are so debilitated when we first see them that they're missing much of school and aren't engaging in typical teenage activities. We offer them the opportunity to participate in a three-week recovery program at our Pediatric Pain Rehabilitation Center Program, which had initially been designed to treat adolescents with chronic pain. The program uses lots of cognitive behavioral therapy techniques, physical therapy, occupational therapy, recreation therapy, and social support. In 2017, we reviewed the results of the first 1,000 adolescents who went through our three-week recovery program; about 200 of them had POTS. Functional ability improved dramatically over the course of the three weeks in the program, and most patients were able to return immediately to full-time school. For even the most compromised POTS patients, recovery of functional ability is to be anticipated.

From all of these helpful but limited reports, we can confidently assert that patients with POTS can potentially fully recover, and some have even recovered within a year of their diagnosis. Of those who keep struggling, improvement is still possible, and good life function is possible even if there are still some symptoms.

👥 LAURA'S PARENTS

The three-week recovery program at Mayo Clinic's Pain Rehabilitation Center (PRC) in Rochester, Minnesota, was the launching pad for Laura's recovery. We had tried coping with POTS on our own for a year before going to PRC. After being diagnosed with POTS, Laura's condition improved. However, after a few months she experienced a routine illness and her POTS symptoms returned in full force and she could not get back on track. It was like she slipped back to square one. She was once again sleeping for long hours and barely attending school.

Our doctor told us about the PRC program and suggested that we explore the program as a next step. When I spoke with the psychologist at PRC in our pre-entry interview she told me the program would give Laura back her life, although not a life she might recognize. But it would definitely help her get her life back.

So Laura will tell you that the three weeks at PRC were very demanding, some of the hardest work she has ever done, but so worth the effort. While in the program Laura learned and practiced essential coping strategies for dealing with her symptoms.

As part of the parent program we learned how to cope with supporting and parenting an unwell teenager. Up until this point we had never had any significant parenting issues with Laura. She was always active, enthusiastic, and busy. Now she was weak, sad, angry, and at home all the time. As parents we were not sure whether to confront some of the behaviors we were seeing or to tiptoe around them so as to not upset things further. This was all new territory for us and we desperately needed help. The PRC parent sessions were invaluable in helping us understand strategies to support and encourage Laura.

At PRC, Laura was with other teenagers who had experienced the same losses she had experienced. Together they supported each other as they navigated their way through the PRC program. To this day they remain close friends and supporters of one another. As parents we found other parents with whom we could converse about some of our daily challenges with parenting unwell teens.

👤 LAURA

After I was diagnosed with POTS, I returned home and implemented the STEPS recovery program into my daily life. However, I got a cold in the beginning of my junior year of high school and my POTS spiraled downhill. I couldn't seem to get back on my feet, and needed a little bit more help. I attended Mayo's three-week Pediatric Pain Rehabilitation Center (PRC) program that summer. PRC helped me learn how to deal with

my symptoms by teaching me lifelong, healthy habits. Throughout my time there, I learned how to fight through my symptoms
by using meditation, deep breathing, and goal-setting. PRC
incorporates physical therapy, occupational therapy, art therapy,
biofeedback, and a variety of other strategies that helped me
take control of my symptoms.

Of course, this doesn't mean that recovery will be easy. One patient
with POTS was asked if she was going to apply for a charity vacation
based on her serious illness. She declined since POTS isn't
life-threatening like cancer. After recovering from POTS, she sadly
developed cancer, unrelated to POTS. She was asked then if she
wanted to go on a charity vacation trip and declined, because cancer
was easier than POTS! She figured that cancer symptoms were fairly
predictable around times of chemotherapy and radiation treatments, but POTS was yucky all of the time with unpredictable times
of worsening. POTS is hard! (She ended up recovering from her
cancer, too.)

Hopefully, with the ideas presented in this book, teens and their
families will be better prepared to deal with chronic fatigue, whatever the cause.

Concluding comments

Wow, we've come a long way together. We've bonded over our shared concern for tired teenagers. We've considered correctable lifestyle factors and treatable medical conditions that can cause fatigue. We've spent time learning to understand the autonomic nervous system and have seen how that has led to additional helpful treatments for postural orthostatic tachycardia syndrome. We put it all into the context of the limits of medical science, and we were reminded that, indeed, most people with POTS do fully recover.

So where does that leave us? Hopefully, we have advanced several steps down the road to recovery. Hopefully, we have a team in place to support ongoing recovery. Hopefully, we see that the answers to chronic fatigue during adolescence are not merely imposed on tired teenagers from doctors, parents, and other people on the outside but that these answers come, in part, from deep within and involve doable hard work.

You've met Laura, who was debilitated with fatigue, and you've shared in her story as she fully recovered. Now, she is succeeding as a medical student. Her parents got to watch her recovery evolve and progress.

👥 LAURA'S PARENTS

Of course there were the obvious signs that recovery was happening. Laura was in school full time. She was exercising regularly without us reminding her to do so. Eventually she had enough energy to drive herself to and from school and to various other events. She was beginning to hang out with friends outside of our home. She was talking about her future and her plans for college. She was preparing for her Senior Violin Recital. We were not talking about her POTS. There was no need to talk about it all the time. She was handling it.

However, the one significant telltale sign that she was improving was the return of her sense of humor. It is not that she lost it completely, but the humorous moments were few and far between early on. Laura was able to find humor in some of the little things that would have previously caused her great despair.

Here is one story …

Laura was in her senior year of high school and she was preparing to attend prom. There was a lot of excitement for this event as it was the first high school dance she would attend since the beginning of her sophomore year. Laura needed her dress altered so we were at a woman's house for her alteration appointment. We had never met this woman before. So here we are in the living room and Laura is in her gown. The woman says to Laura, "I need you to stand really still so I can get this hem just right." Laura looks at me with complete horror as both she and I know she cannot stand still. Laura is always moving to and fro to keep the blood from pooling in her feet, to keep from fainting. But today Laura has decided to give it her best shot. Within about 30 seconds of standing completely still, Laura turns to me and says, "Mom, I don't feel …" and with that she faints flat out on this woman's (whom we just met) living room floor, in her beautiful gown. A few moments later Laura starts to come around and this sweet lady leans over Laura and says, "Girl, you need to eat more greens!" Laura laughed all the way home from that appointment. We still laugh about this and we always say if eating greens was all that it took … and then we laugh some more.

Laura's sense of humor was an indication to us that she understood her POTS, she knew how to handle her symptoms, and she was going to enjoy life despite it.

It's been a long journey for Laura and her family, but Laura is now healthy and thriving. It's been a long journey to prepare this book, too. I started planning the book more than a decade ago, and it has been ripening since. Along the way, science has advanced and literally thousands of my tired teenage patients have made good recoveries. My hope is that this book will help others follow their examples of success.

I've tried to keep this book conversational, and I haven't listed academic references to medical articles. But I've put clues of authors and topics of papers in this book so that you, if you want to see all of the data, can find articles and resources online, either through a regular search engine or at PubMed.

And the conversation continues! Feel free to share your stories and ideas with me at TiredTeenagers@gmail.com. As medicine continues to advance, maybe there will someday be a new edition of this book that incorporates some of the things you'll tell me.

Let's wrap this book up with comments from the mother of another of the patients I saw, a teenager who came because she was tired and then went home to get better. Hopefully each of us can have the same positive experience, even without needing to make a long trip to Minnesota.

> I am just stunned at the difference in my daughter
> since we have returned home.
> She is exercising daily without prompting,
> following her regimen exactly,
> and is back to school and going places every day.
> I could go on and on. It is just amazing and such a joy.
> If there is one thing I could pin the improvement on,
> I believe that our trip gave her back HOPE!

May you, too, be filled with hope. May you follow your recovery regimen exactly, exercising, going to school, and socializing. Be amazed! You, too, can recover!

Index

tiredness in teens. See chronic fatigue

TSH (thyroid stimulating hormone), 39

U

ulcerative colitis, 42
urinary problems, 118
urinary tract infections (UTIs), 41

V

vertigo, 103, 105
vitamin D deficiency, 175
VO2 max (maximum oxygen uptake), 66–68, 71–73

W

weight appropriate to height, 73